A PRACTICAL INTRODUCTION TO

HOMEOPATHY

LIZ CHARLES

Acknowledgments
Photography: Charles Walker Picture Library p. 10, 11, 12, 13 and 15

Published in 2002 by Caxton Editions
20 Bloomsbury Street
London WC1B 3JH
a member of the Caxton Publishing Group

© 2002 Caxton Publishing Group

Designed and produced for Caxton Editions
by Open Door Limited, Rutland, United Kingdom

Editing: Mary Morton
Setting: Jane Booth
Digital Imagery © copyright 2002 PhotoDisc Inc.

Title: A Practical Introduction to Homeopathy
ISBN: 1 84067 304 4

IMPORTANT NOTICE:
This book is not intended to be a substitute for medical advice or treatment.
Any person with a condition requiring medical attention should consult a qualified
medical practitioner or therapist.

A PRACTICAL INTRODUCTION TO
HOMEOPATHY

LIZ CHARLES

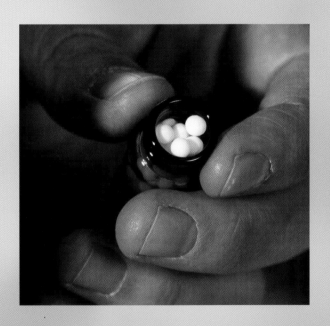

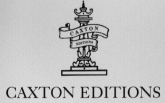

CAXTON EDITIONS

CONTENTS

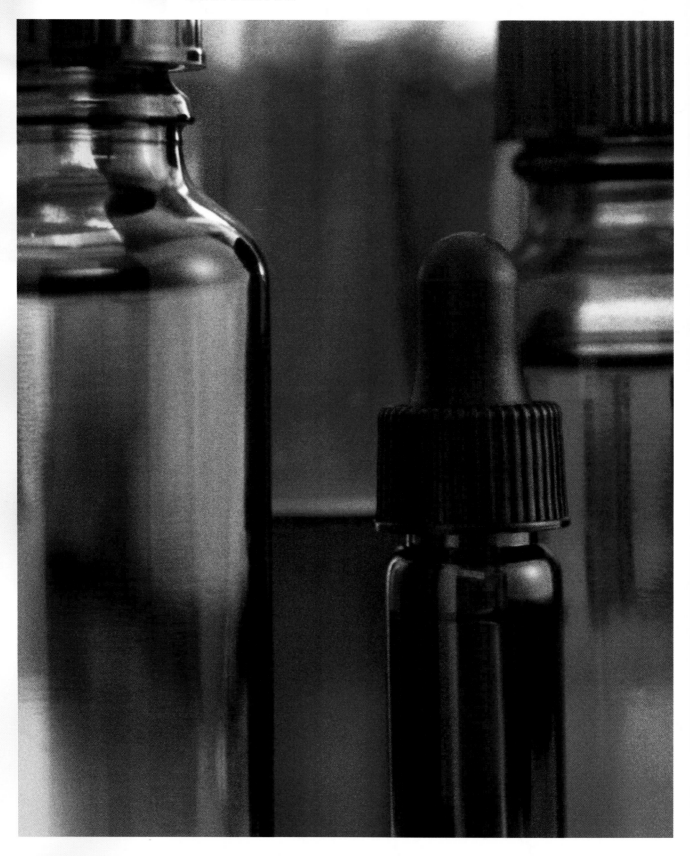

CONTENTS

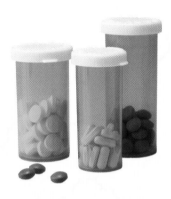
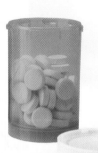

INTRODUCTION

Below: this book aims to offer a balanced and comprehensive view of the homeopathy

Traditionally, Western medicine aims to cure an illness with a drug that has the opposite effect to the symptoms. Homeopathy stands that tradition on its head. It treats the disease by administering minute doses of agents that, in a healthy person, would actually produce the symptoms of the illness.

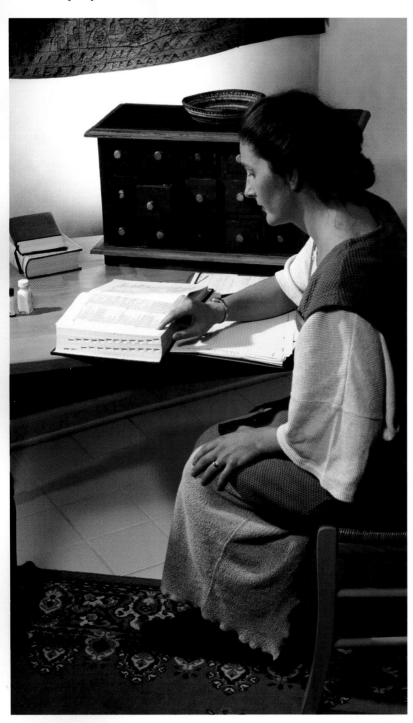

This is treating like with like. The nearest equivalent to be found in modern medical practice is vaccination, where the cowpox virus is used against smallpox. Injected into a healthy person, the virus stimulates the body to produce its own antibodies and hence immunity against the disease.

So it is with homeopathy.

This book aims to offer a balanced and comprehensive view of the subject, explaining the background to homeopathy and how the layman can safely use it.

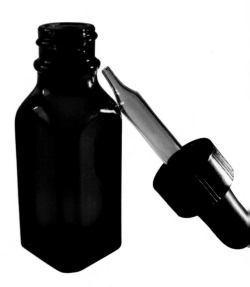

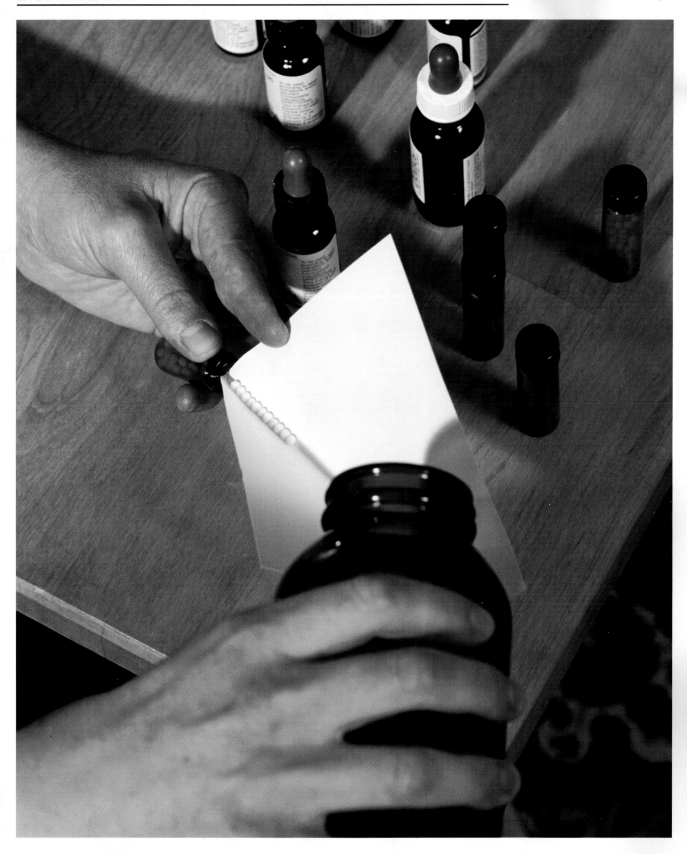

HOMEOPATHY

WHAT IS HOMEOPATHY?

Homeopathy is a long-established form of complementary medicine, distinguished by its belief in "the potent force of the minimum dose". The name itself is derived from two Greek words – *homoios* (meaning similar) and *pathos* (meaning suffering).

THE HOLISTIC APPROACH

You will notice one big difference between a homeopathic practitioner and the usual GP.

Below: modern homeopaths seek to stimulate this natural resistance to disease by prescribing according to the Law of Similars.

The homeopath studies and treats the whole person, whereas modern medicine often considers only the symptoms presented or that part of the body in which they occur. However, an increasing number of medical doctors now acknowledge the benefits of homeopathy. Some have themselves qualified in the therapy and others are happy to refer their patients to a homeopathic practitioner.

THE VITAL FORCE

During the 17th century, it was fashionable to believe that the body was regulated by a "Vital Force". This theory – known as "vitalism" – maintained that symptoms of disease were an indication that this mystical inner force was fighting infection.

Nowadays, we refer to this reaction as the auto-immune system. Modern homeopaths seek to stimulate this natural resistance to disease by prescribing according to the Law of Similars.

LIKE WILL CURE LIKE

Homeopathy is based on the belief that "like will cure like". In other words, a minute dose of a substance that causes similar symptoms to those suffered by the patient will stimulate the healing powers of their own body and cure their condition.

This is known as the Law of Similars – and could perhaps be described as "a hair of the dog that bit you".

TABLETS OR POWDERS

Homeopathic remedies come in powder or tablet form or as tinctures. They are stocked by most pharmacies and health stores and no prescription is needed. The homeopathic approach is essentially gentle and, in marked contrast to some medically prescribed treatments, there are no side-effects.

COMMON SENSE

One big advantage of homeopathic remedies is that they are readily available and are known to be absolutely safe. This means that most everyday ailments can be treated without spending hours in a doctor's surgery waiting for them to scribble a prescription.

However, common sense should prevail. For example, homeopathy can effectively treat the common cold but, should the infection move to the chest or worsen in any way, a doctor must be consulted. Don't even consider increasing the strength of the remedy you are taking. Always remember the basic tenet of homeopathic treatment – the potent force of the minimum dose.

SERIOUS CONDITIONS

Although homeopathy can be used to treat all manner of ailments, it must be clearly understood that serious conditions need the attention of a qualified homeopath.

If you are unfortunate enough to suffer from a serious illness such as ME, asthma, angina, psoriasis, multiple sclerosis or any other severe problem, see your GP and ask them to refer you to a professional homeopath. You will obtain relief much more quickly in this way. Attempting self-treatment for any serious and/or long-standing condition will only prolong your suffering.

TRIED AND TESTED

Homeopathy has been widely used in medical practice for more than 200 years. During that time it has become accepted as a safe, gentle and effective method of treatment for innumerable medical conditions. It is widely accepted by the medical profession and is one of the few complementary therapies to be available from the NHS.

Below: homeopathic remedies are readily available and are known to be absolutely safe.

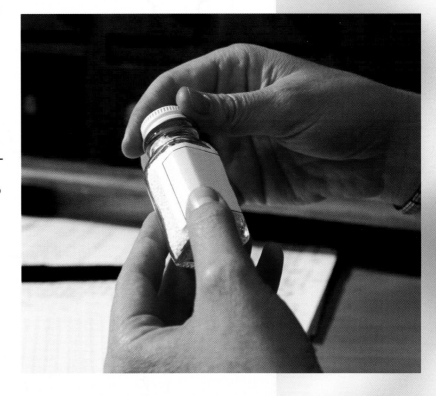

HOW HOMEOPATHY BEGAN

The homeopathic Law of Similars (that like will cure like) originated in the fifth century BC with the Greek physician Hippocrates. This concept was in direct contrast to the Law of Contraries, practised by most medical men of the time. As a result, the idea received only limited attention.

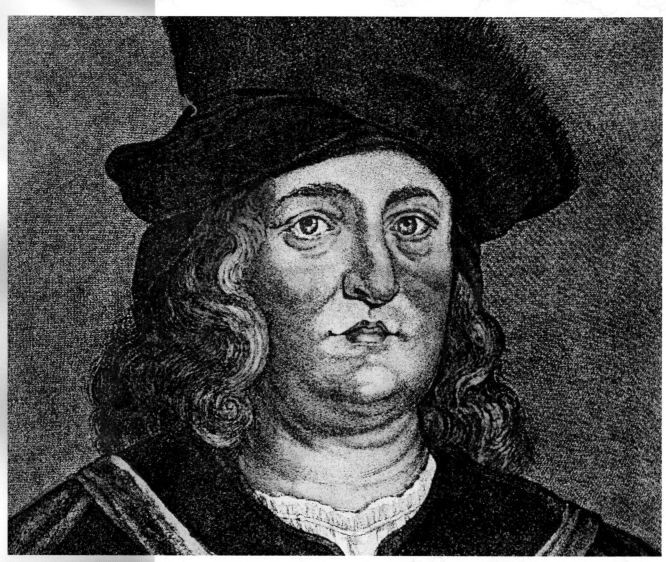

Above: the Swiss physician Philippus Aureolus Paracelsus (1493–1541).

Further medical developments came through the Romans who, in the first to fifth centuries AD, set great store by the use of herbs.

European medicine remained static for some considerable time. It was not until many centuries later that further progress was made. The man largely responsible for this was the Swiss physician Philippus Aureolus Paracelsus (1493–1541).

THE DOCTRINE OF SIGNATURES

It was Paracelsus who initiated the revival of the DOCTRINE OF SIGNATURES. This ancient Greek theory claims that the external appearance of a plant is, in fact, God's signature. It follows therefore that the healing properties possessed by a plant, and the ailments it can be expected to treat, are clearly indicated by its shape and colour.

The famous English herbalist Nicholas Culpeper (1616–1654) agreed with this theory. He was referring to the Lesser Celandine (Ranunculus Ficaria) commonly known as Pilewort when in *The Compleat Herbal*, published in 1649, he wrote:

> *"The virtue of an herb may be known by its signature as plainly appears in this. For if you dig up the root of it, you shall perceive the perfect imagine of the disease which they commonly call the piles."*

GREAT OAKS FROM LITTLE ACORNS...

Paracelsus is often called "the father of chemistry" and he was probably the first physician ever to recognise the importance of precise dosage. He it was who claimed that "it all depends on the dose whether a poison is a poison or not".

This conviction, and his support for the belief that "like will cure like," established Paracelsus as one of the pioneers in the form of treatment that eventually became known as homeopathy. James Compton Burnett (1840–1901), an eminent British homeopath, declared that: "Paracelsus planted the acorn from which the mighty oak of homeopathy has grown."

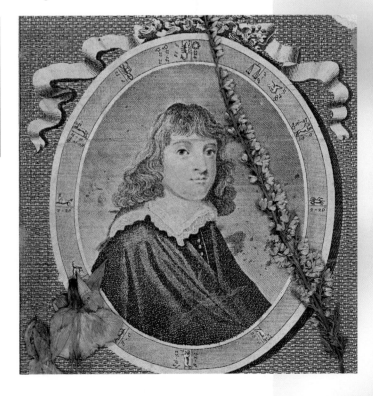

Below: English herbalist Nicholas Culpeper (1616–1654)

THE AMAZING DR HAHNEMANN

At the end of the 18th century, the health of the citizens in most European countries was poor. This was largely due to three factors:

malnutrition;

the spread of infection in overcrowded newly industrialised cities;

deplorably low standards of public hygiene.

These were the conditions when Samuel Hahnemann (1755–1843) started his medical career.

By any standards, Hahnemann was a remarkable young man. At the age of 20 he entered the University of Leipzig to study medicine. He was already fluent in eight languages. He qualified as a Doctor of Medicine in 1779 and married almost immediately. Inevitably, he soon had a family to support and turned to writing in an effort to supplement his income.

Below: Samuel Hahnemann (1755–1843).

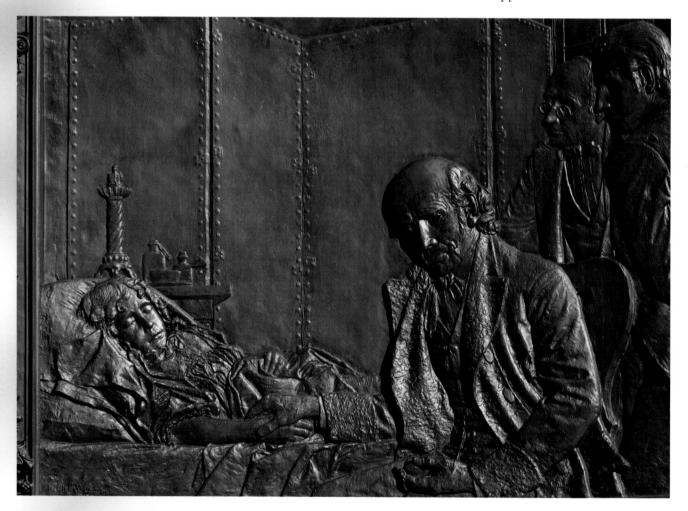

DISILLUSION

As soon as he set up his medical practice, Hahnemann became disillusioned with the drastic and often harmful "remedies" employed by even the most eminent physicians of the day.

He was particularly disturbed by the conditions in which mentally disturbed patients were kept. Most were restrained in chains, subjected to violence and abuse from their "carers", and tormented by the public who were allowed to view them from a safe distance.

Hahnemann wrote:
"...these sufferers deserve only pity..."

Primitive treatments such as blood-letting were commonplace and most doctors considered this an essential part of any treatment. They were less than impressed, too, when Hahnemann claimed that some doctors actually experimented on their patients, mixing as many as 10 drugs at a time.

His articles were savagely critical of such practices. He himself always used drugs singly and would not repeat the dose until he was sure of the patient's reaction.

In those days, a young doctor who concerned himself with the patient's housing and diet was regarded as more than slightly mad. This opinion of him was strengthened when, in 1790, Hahnemann began to experiment on himself.

At this time, he was translating *A Treatise on Materia* MEDICA by Dr William Cullen. In this book, the learned doctor claimed that Cinchona bark, which contained the astringent quinine, was effective in the treatment of "the intermittent fever" (now known as malaria.) Hahnemann did not believe this and set out to disprove Cullen's theory.

Below: primitive treatments such as blood-letting were commonplace and most doctors considered this an essential part of any treatment.

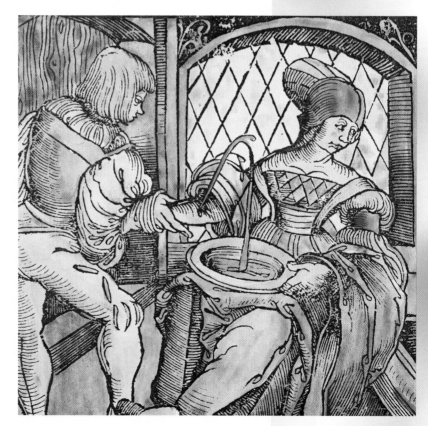

TESTING

Although he was perfectly healthy and not suffering from any illness, he dosed himself with Cinchona – and immediately began to develop the fever symptoms. As soon as he stopped taking the remedy, the symptoms lessened. When he took another dose of Cinchona, they recurred.

He wrote:

> "This paroxysm lasted two or three hours each time, and recurred if I repeated this dose, not otherwise; I discontinued it and was in good health."

He repeated the experiment with several volunteers, all of whom had the same results.

At this time, it was generally accepted that the sole purpose of medical treatment was to provide a prescription that would relieve the patient's symptoms. Hahnemann's experiments with Cincho∆na bark stood this theory on its head. Administering to a healthy patient the drug believed to cure "the intermittent fever" actually produced the symptoms of the disease.

RESEARCH GROUP

When Hahnemann's discovery became known, he was surprised and delighted to be contacted by other like-minded physicians. They, too, were disenchanted with contemporary medical practice and were eager to learn new methods. A small research group was formed. For six years, the doctors experimented upon themselves by taking different drugs. They kept detailed records of the symptoms these drugs produced.

THE START OF HOMEOPATHY

This then was how homeopathy began. Noting the patient's symptoms, Hahnemann prescribed medicine that had produced similar reactions in himself or one of his colleagues. Almost invariably, the patient was cured – sometimes after the very first dose.

INITIAL SUCCESS

Because homeopathic treatment was so obviously beneficial, particularly in treating infectious disorders, it swiftly became popular. This was a process undoubtedly aided by the various serious epidemics – cholera, scarlet fever and typhoid fever – so prevalent at that time. Homeopathy alleviated the suffering of thousands of people and practitioners were much in demand.

PERSECUTION

Despite the popularity and success of homeopathy with the patients themselves, the anti-homeopathy movement grew. Doctors distrusted any new approach and were afraid they would lose financially. Apothecaries, realising that homeopathic treatments were considerably cheaper than the drugs they dispensed, were equally suspicious. Facing such organised antagonism, homeopaths began to experience many forms of persecution. Court cases, mostly engineered by rival doctors, resulted in heavy fines and even imprisonment, with resulting damaging publicity.

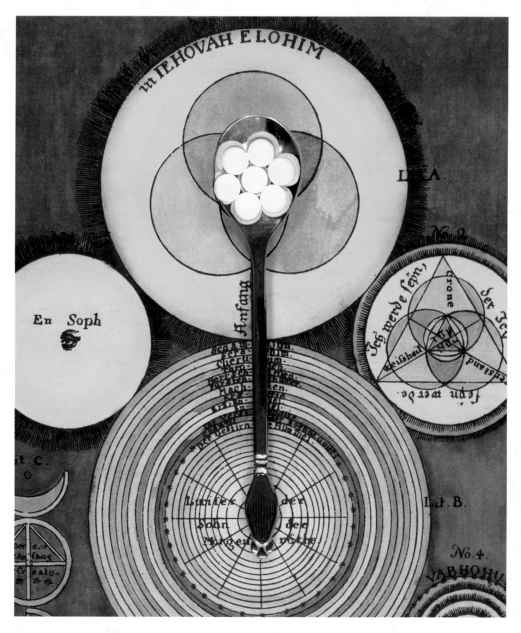

Left: pilules in a dispensing spoon, overlaid on a plate based on the alchemical work of Franciscus van Helmont.

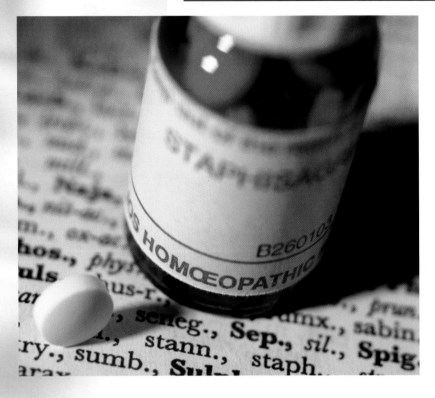

Above: unlike some alternative therapies, too, homeopathy has a reputable and solid background.

19TH CENTURY DISCOVERIES

When, towards the end of the 19th century, the discoveries of Lister and Pasteur were announced, public interest in homeopathy waned. Sulphonamides were the 'in' thing. Medical treatment was again directed towards treatment of the disease itself. The homeopathic principle of treating the individual rather than the illness became discredited. Even so, it has been estimated that at this time more than 400 million people worldwide were receiving homeopathic treatment.

CLINICAL TRIALS

It was not until the 1980s that any real clinical trials of homeopathy were embarked upon in Britain. The popularity of drugs and the influence of the huge companies manufacturing them have, until recently, handicapped funding of any such research. There has also been a tendency to regard the success of homeopathic treatment as "the placebo effect" – suggesting that the remedies work because the patient expects them to. More recent investigations, though – in 1991, 1996 and 1997 – indicate that this is not so.

CURRENT INTEREST

Homeopathy has obviously benefited from the surge of public interest in complementary medicine. Unlike some alternative therapies, too, homeopathy has a reputable and solid background. An increasing number of medical professionals are also qualified homeopaths. The treatment is available at several homeopathic hospitals and is available at many NHS Trusts.

Alarmed by the sometimes drastic side-effects of conventional medicine, many people are seeking the more gentle ways of homeopathy. Also to be considered is the rising cost of healthcare. Homeopathic medicines are invariably cheaper than drugs and, for this very reason, may be more readily available from the stretched resources of the NHS.

As we have established, homeopathy differs from allopathic medicine in that it treats the whole person, not just the symptoms presented. Where medical doctors regard the symptoms themselves as the illness, homeopaths believe that they are indications of the body's attempts to heal itself. The three main principles established by Dr Hahnemann in the 19th century still hold good. These are

Below: treating the whole person

1	*The Law of Similars*
2	*The minimum dose*
3	*Treating the whole person*

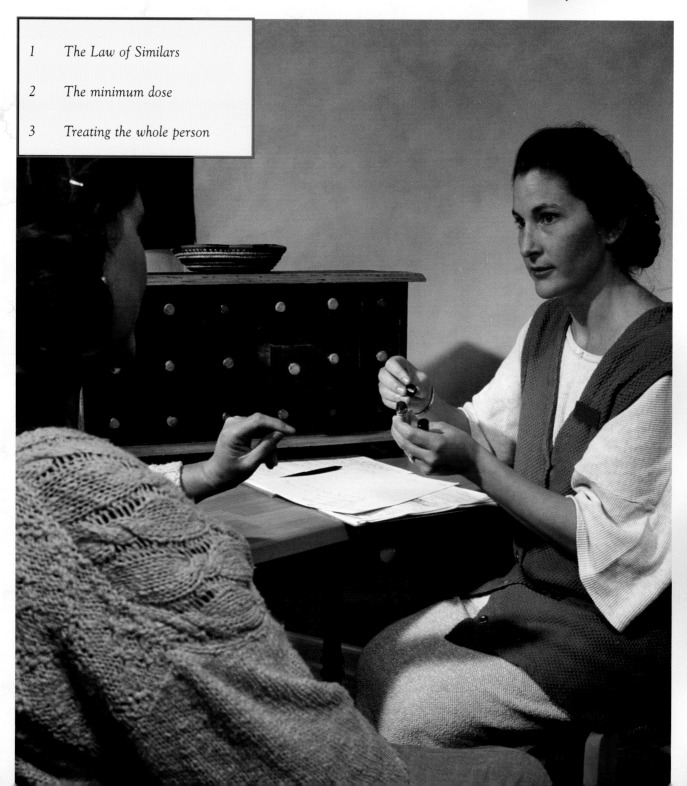

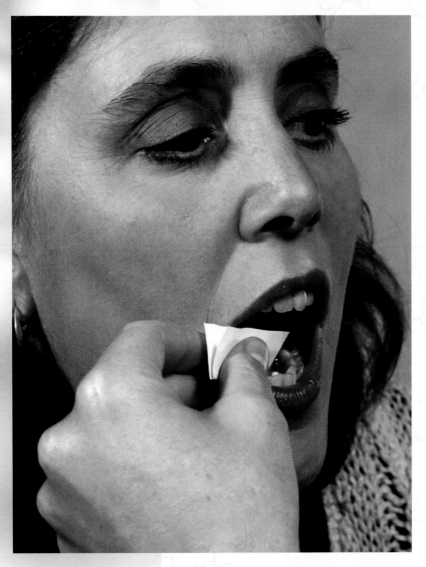

Above: homeopathic remedies come in different strengths or potencies, the most common of which are 6c. and 30c.

He believed that if a large dose of a certain substance can produce symptoms of disease in a healthy person, a minute amount of it would cure similar symptoms in the person who is sick.

As an example, the symptoms of Belladonna poisoning are very much the same as those of scarlet fever. Thus Belladonna would be the remedy selected to treat the disease.

THE MINIMUM DOSE

Some of the drugs from which homeopathic remedies are made are extremely strong or even poisonous. Hahnemann used only very small amounts of such substances in his prescriptions. Even so, his patients still suffered what he described as "aggravations" – or, in modern language, side-effects.

After a number of experiments, he discovered a method of preparation that he called "potentisation", whereby extreme dilution of the active ingredient actually enhanced its curative properties. From then on, this is how Hahnemann treated his patients – and the "aggravations" ceased.

THE LAW OF SIMILARS

Hahnemann himself gave a succinct explanation of this law in his book *Organon of Practical Medicine*.
He wrote:

> *To achieve a gentle and lasting cure, always choose a drug capable of provoking a disease similar to the one it is to cure.*

POTENCIES

Homeopathic remedies come in different strengths or potencies, the most common of which are 6c. and 30c. Potentisation occurs when the remedy is not only diluted, but also vigorously shaken at each stage of the preparation. This process, according to Hahnemann, gradually releases the potency of the substance. In consequence, the healing effect becomes stronger and longer lasting.

For self-treatment, much depends on the type of complaint from which you are suffering. If it is physical, the 6c. potency is best. The 30c. potency may be more effective if you have severe emotional problems. If in doubt, enquire at the pharmacy where you buy the remedy.

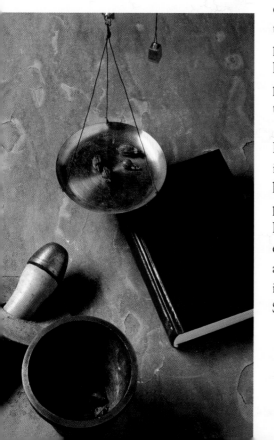

TREATING THE INDIVIDUAL

The third of Hahnemann's principles concerned the treatment of the whole person, not merely the symptoms they are exhibiting. He believed that the remedies he prescribed worked because they stimulated what he called the Vital Force.

This was his term for the healing energy that exists in every human being. It has many names – in China it is called chi and in India the word is prana. The existence of this inner power has been acknowledged for thousands of years. It is this Vital Force that maintains our physical, mental and emotional health. Any imbalance of this force can result in illness.

As we have already seen, Hahnemann carefully prescribed his remedies for the specific needs of each individual patient. He believed that in so doing, he was able to strengthen that patient's Vital Force and stimulate their body's healing powers.

Despite this emphasis on the importance of the individual, however, it is possible to classify most patients into "constitutional types". Each type appears to possess certain emotional, physical and mental traits and it is these that the practitioner is investigating at a first consultation. See page 22 for more information.

Left: some of the drugs from which homeopathic remedies are made are extremely strong or even poisonous. Hahnemann used only very small amounts of such substances in his prescriptions.

THE LAW OF CURE

Practitioners believe that, in addition to the three principles detailed above, there is also a Law of Cure. This states that:

The remedy starts at the top and works down the body.

It works from inside the body outwards.

It goes from major to minor organs.

Symptoms clear in reverse order to that in which they appear.

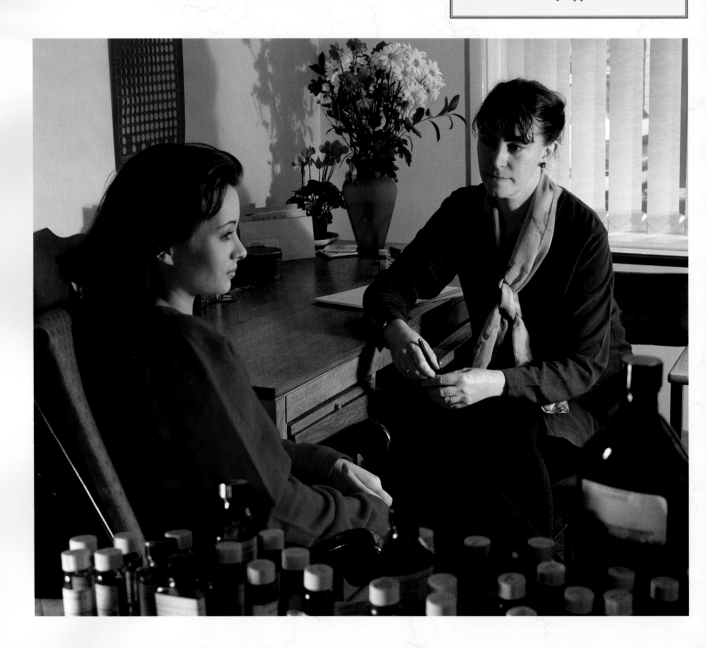

One of the basic principles of homeopathy is that it is gentle and non-invasive. Remedies are known to be perfectly safe and are readily available over the counter at pharmacies and health shops. It is not surprising, therefore, that so many people decide to treat themselves, perhaps being guided by one of the many books on the subject.

This is not always a wise decision. Although the remedies themselves are harmless, it is essential to first consider the gravity of the ailment being treated. A course of self-prescribed homeopathic treatment could well be unsuccessful when dealing with severe illness. Furthermore, the condition could worsen due to delay in seeking qualified treatment.

MINOR AILMENTS

A number of minor ailments and injuries can be safely treated by self-prescription. Generally speaking, an illness can be considered as minor if it does not radically affect your lifestyle. Thus, mild indigestion may be uncomfortable but it is unlikely to be dangerous. Flatulence can usually be relieved by the use of Carbo veg. (commonly known as charcoal). However, if the symptoms persist, if you experience severe pain, or if you vomit blood, you should consult a doctor immediately.

In fact, the most sensible procedure is to always consult a doctor or a homeopathic practitioner about any symptom that persists for more than a week. If they assure you that there is nothing to worry about, then you can try treating yourself with homeopathy. Alternatively, your doctor may advise you as to which homeopathic remedies will be most suitable, or guide you towards a practitioner.

FINDING A THERAPIST

If your doctor is unable to give you the name of a reputable therapist, you would be well advised to contact one of the recognised homeopathic organisations. (See Appendix at the end of this book.) It is better to do this than to pick out a name at random from the *Yellow Pages* or from your local newspaper. If, for any reason, you need to contact a homeopath urgently, then at least ensure that he/she is a member of a professional association.

Far left: if your doctor is unable to give you the name of a reputable therapist, you would be well advised to contact one of the recognised homeopathic organisations.

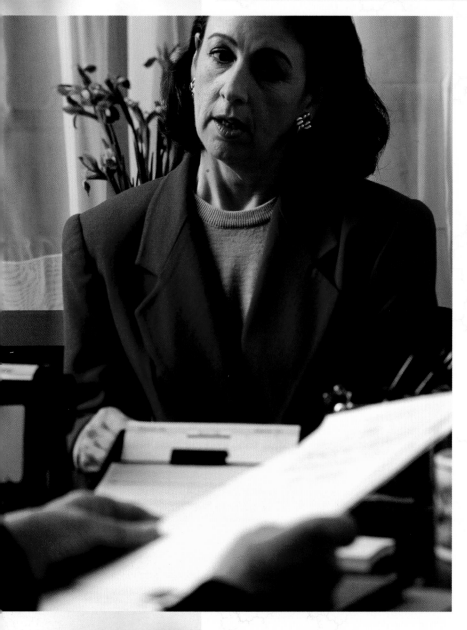

Above: be prepared to answer a great many questions.

consultation will take much longer than a visit to your GP. Be prepared to answer a great many questions. Remember that homeopathy is an holistic treatment. That being so, the practitioner needs to learn about every aspect of you as a person, your life and your habits. Allow at least an hour, probably longer, for your initial consultation.

TELL THE TRUTH

Remember, too, that it is essential to be truthful. If, for example, you are a heavy smoker, then admit it. If you give misleading or inaccurate information to your practitioner, you are effectively handicapping your own chances of being healed.

ASSESSING THE PATIENT

During their assessment of you, their new patient, the practitioner will ask many questions. These will probably be grouped under half a dozen headings, such as:

Your physical condition

Your mental and emotional well-being

Your past life

Your medical history

Your lifestyle

Your home and work environment

THE FIRST CONSULTATION

Having contacted your homeopath and made an appointment to see them, what should you expect at the first consultation?

Certainly you should remember to allow plenty of time. A homeopathic

PHYSICAL CONDITION

They will probably begin by asking for an exact description of your symptoms, how and when they began and how they affect you. Because of time limitation, most GPs prefer you to be brief and to the point. In marked contrast, the homeopathic practitioner will encourage you to relate even the most minute and apparently irrelevant details of the way you feel.

They will ask you to step on the scales to check your weight. Then come some searching questions.

How much exercise do you take?
How well do you sleep?

What sort of food do you eat?
Are there any foods that "disagree" with you?

Do you smoke, drink alcohol or use drugs?

How much leisure time do you have?
How do you spend it?

MENTAL AND EMOTIONAL STATE

The questions asked under this category will be mainly concerned with your temperament and personality.

Do you consider yourself to be a basically happy person?

Are you self-reliant or do you feel inadequate to cope with daily life?

How do you cope with stress – in an emergency or over a long period?

Are you demonstrative or do you find it difficult to express your emotions?

Do you have any religious or spiritual convictions? How much do they affect your way of life?

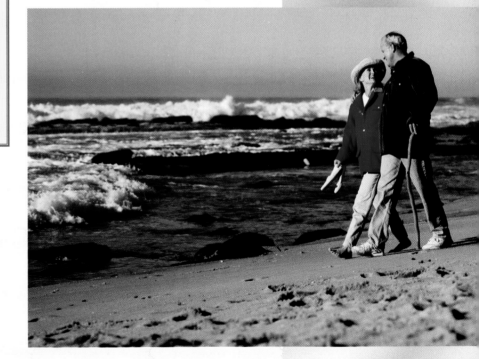

Below: how much leisure time to do you have? How do you spend it?

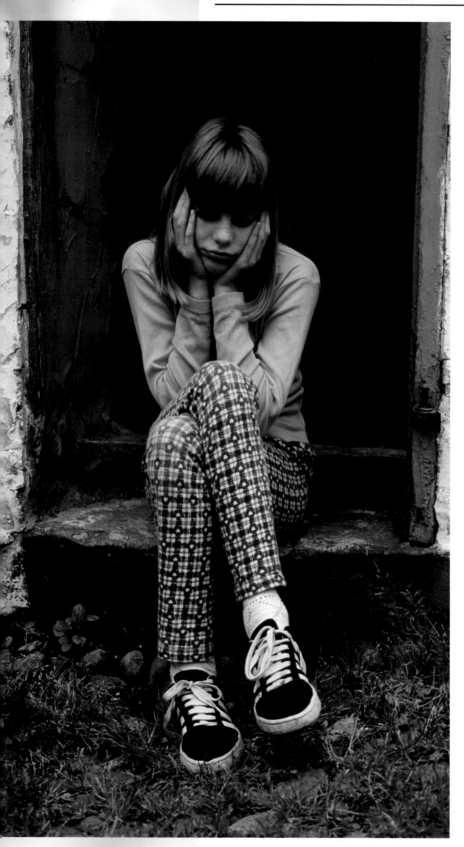

PAST LIFE

Here again, you should not hesitate to "let your hair down" in answer to the questions you will be asked. Do understand that it is the events and experiences of your past life that have shaped the person you are now.

Did you have a happy childhood? If not, why not?

What was your position in the family?

Were there any traumatic family events – parents' death or divorce, severe illness, accidents, etc.?

How many times did your family move house?

Were you happy at school? If not, why not?

Were you aware of any family financial problems?

MEDICAL HISTORY

The practitioner will want to know about your own medical history, but will also need to be aware of any possible inherited tendencies.

What illnesses, injuries or surgery have you experienced and when?

What is the medical history of your family? Does anyone suffer from heart trouble, cancer, etc.?

Does your family have any history of mental problems?

Is there any family tendency towards allergies, hay fever, etc.?

Do you have regular medical checks?

What is the family attitude to health – positive or tending towards hypochondria?

LIFESTYLE

This section covers your life as it is now – and you may well be asked some questions about how you would like to change it.

Do you live alone? If so, are you happy to do so?

How good is your relationship with your family – partner, children, siblings and parents?

Are you happy in your work? If not, why not?

Do you have any financial problems? What are your plans for the future? Are you taking any definite steps towards achieving them?

Do you feel that you have adequate personal space – time to yourself for recreation, interests, socialising, etc.?

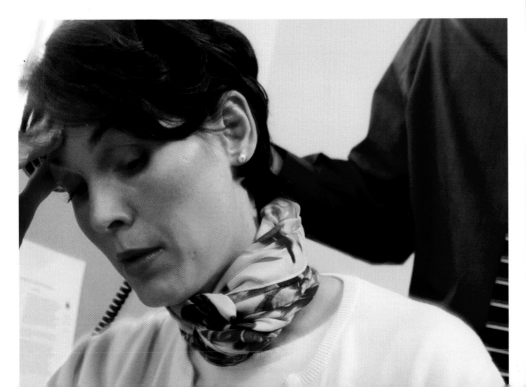

Far left: did you have a happy childhood? If not, why not?

Left: are you happy in your work? If not, why not?

Right: do you have a long journey to your work place? Are you stressed by commuting?

ENVIRONMENT

This is a wide-ranging section and will cover a variety of topics. Some of the questions may even concern your personal attitude towards ecology, pollution and similar topics.

> *Are you happy with the place you live? If not, why not?*
>
> *Are you happy with the place you work? If not, why not?*
>
> *Do you have a long journey to your work place? Are you stressed by commuting?*
>
> *Do you have a fairly regular daily routine or do you seem to spend your whole life on the run?*

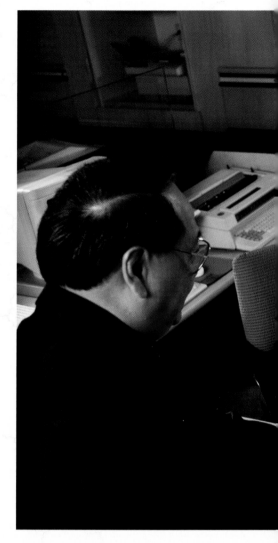

These are merely a few examples of the questions your homeopathic practitioner may ask you. There will probably be many more. The aim is to create a complete picture of you as a person – your physical, mental and emotional state, your attitudes to various aspects of your life, your likes and dislikes, any personal idiosyncrasies you may have.

YOU ARE UNIQUE

It is a truism that there is nobody else in the world exactly like you. One of the most fascinating aspects of life is the realisation that though human beings may appear to be basically similar, each one of us is unique. For this reason, the remedy prescribed for your ailments must also be unique – individual to you.

It is extremely unlikely that any two people will be given the same prescription. Even if the symptoms presented are identical, the patients concerned will be totally different personalities and the remedies prescribed will differ.

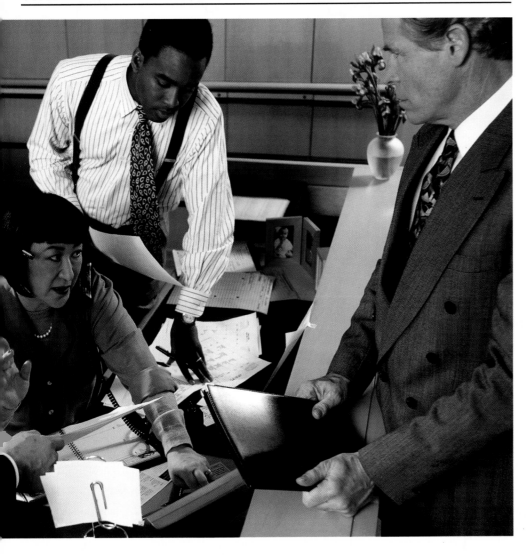

AFTER THE FIRST ASSESSMENT

Your consultation with a homeopath is likely to be the first of several. You will probably be asked to agree to a series of follow-up visits, often with several weeks between interviews. Don't imagine that the need for further investigation means that your problem is particularly serious or dangerous. The intention is for your practitioner to hold a watching brief on the progress you are making.

You may find that the remedies suggested will change, as various aspects of your problems are resolved. Homeopathy is an holistic treatment, dealing not only with the symptoms but the underlying causes for them.

Trust your practitioner to provide you with the best, most effective and safest treatment.

HOMEOPATHIC CLASSIFICATIONS

TYPE CASTING

The searching questions you will be asked on your first visit to a homeopath will enable them to discover your constitutional type.

> *What does this mean?*

As we have already explained, a homeopathic practitioner treats the whole person, not merely the symptoms. In assessing a new patient, they take into consideration absolutely everything that constitutes that person. (See previous section *Visiting a Practitioner*.)

Various homeopathic types are said to have in common a number of distinctive physical, mental and emotional traits. This is why it is unusual for two people to be prescribed the same remedy, even though they present the same symptoms.

Hahnemann himself was the first to realise that certain types of people seem to have an affinity for a specific drug and therefore respond positively to it. For example – Pulsatilla has been used since Roman times to treat tearfulness. Hence, if you tend to cry easily and suffer from colds, eye infections and PMS, you are likely to be classified as a Pulsatilla type.

Below: various homeopathic types are said to have in common a number of distinctive physical, mental and emotional traits.

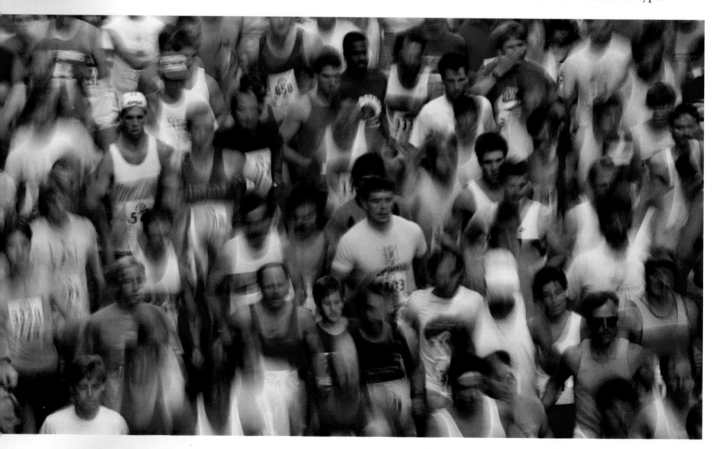

WHICH TYPE ARE YOU?

Argent. nit.
These people are extroverts. Usually cheerful, they are easily motivated and are often found in highly pressurised jobs. They tend to suffer from nervous problems and anxiety and are always in a hurry. They are extremely sensitive to heat, with a tendency to phobias, and digestive problems.

Arsen. alb.
If any of your friends are perfectionists, they are likely to be classified as Arsen. alb. types. These people are always on the go, are extremely ambitious, and need constant reassurance about their health. They may have breathing difficulties and headaches and are particularly susceptible to food poisoning.

Calc. carb.
This type is usually quiet, cautious and often overweight. They can be somewhat obsessive and become extremely agitated when faced with any form of cruelty. Their circulation is slow and they tend to suffer from perspiration problems. Prone to constipation, they often suffer from pains in the joints and dental problems. Women of this type are particularly susceptible to gynaecological ailments.

Graphites
These people seem quite unable to make up their minds about anything. They prefer action to discussion and are generally regarded as helpful, reliable people. Lethargy can be a problem for them, and they are particularly subject to skin eruptions. Headaches also trouble them – usually on the left side of the head.

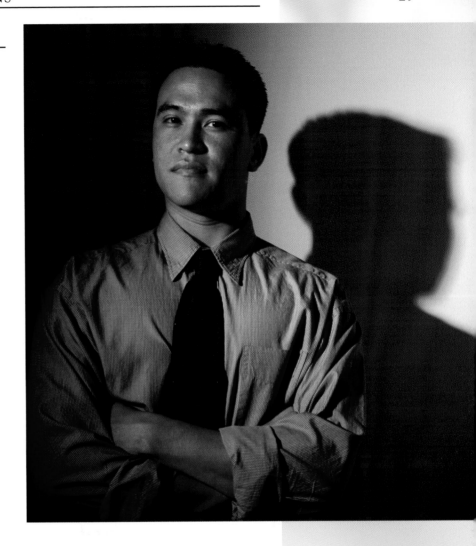

Above: Arsen. alb. people are always on the go and extremely ambitious.

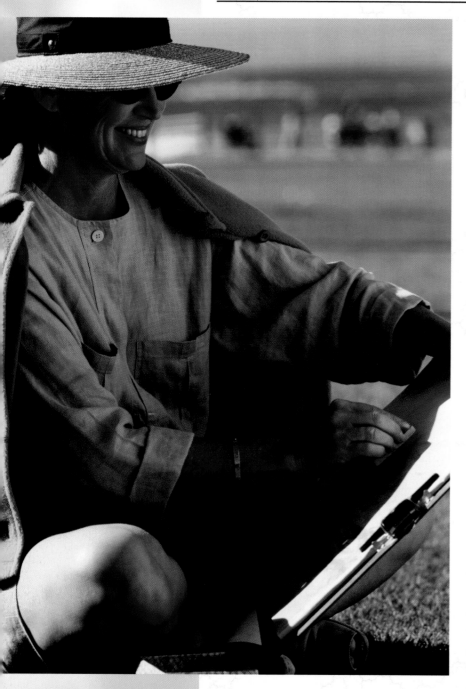

Above: your Lachesis friends will almost certainly be extremely creative.

Ignatia

People of the Ignatia type are often dark-haired women, extremely emotional, artistic and full of idealistic dreams. They are the "clinging" type and the breakdown of a marriage or close relationship will have a devastating effect. Mood swings are common here and they tend to indulge in self-pity. Other typical common weaknesses include hysteria and other nervous problems, sore throats and digestive upsets. They are particularly sensitive to pain and – oddly – are often afraid of birds.

Lachesis

Your Lachesis friends will almost certainly be extremely creative – with a tendency to blow up if they meet with any opposition. They will also be talkative, dogmatic and surprisingly perceptive. They have a tendency to burn the candle at both ends and this may be the reason for the marked fluctuations in their energy levels. There are times when they find it difficult to control their emotions. Typical problems include varicose veins, nervous disorders and such conditions as angina. Women of the Lachesis type may have problems with premenstrual syndrome (PMS) and during the menopause.

Lycopodium

Lycopodium types are noticeably intolerant of illness, including their own. They have to feel very poorly indeed before they will admit to it and even then will be reluctant to seek help. Their lack of confidence is often hidden behind a façade of sarcasm and arrogance with the result that other people tend to be wary of them. Despite their reclusive attitude, they suffer from anxiety and this may cause the digestive upsets they experience. This type of person may suffer from dyslexia, insomnia, kidney stones and chest problems.

Merc. sol.

These people are highly introverted, quick-tempered and easily offended. They desperately need stability and this is reflected in their desire for a well-ordered existence. This conventional front serves to conceal their inner sense of urgency. At times, the feelings they are trying to hide can burst out in an explosion of rage. Merc. sol. types are particularly susceptible to respiratory illnesses, and to problems with the mouth and throat. Women of this type often suffer from thrush.

Below: Merc. sol. people are highly introverted, quick tempered and easily offended.

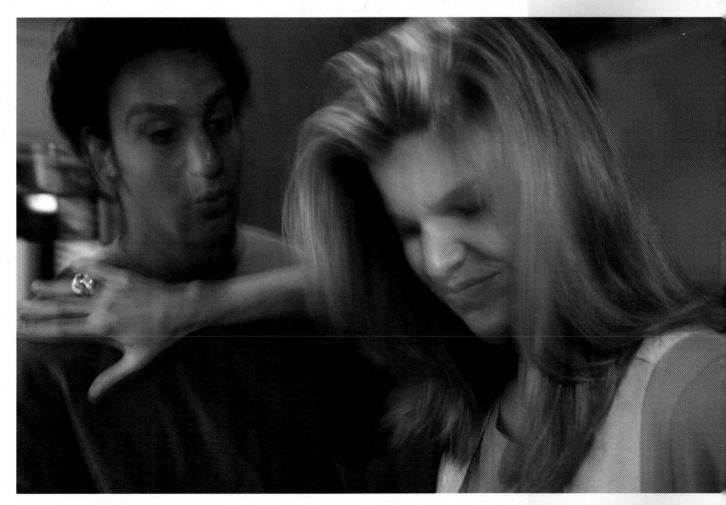

Nat. mur.

Nat. mur. people are highly sensitive and introspective, sometimes repressing their emotions more than is wise. One result of this is that they give the impression of being totally self-reliant. In fact, they long to make friends but are held back by their inhibitions and lack of confidence in social situations. Nat. mur. types will catch any cold that's going, but reject sympathy however ill they feel. Many of the ailments from which these people suffer are caused by their own introverted personalities.

Nux vomica

Most of the workaholics you know will be Nux vomica types. Highly-strung and impatient, they are the entrepreneurs of society and thrive on challenge. These people work hard – and play with equal energy. In fact, they tend to go over the top in every aspect of their lives. They eat too much, drink too heavily, have high sex drives, and may well indulge in drugs. Not surprisingly, their lifestyle results in a variety of health problems, including insomnia, headaches, tension, irritable bowel syndrome and ulcers.

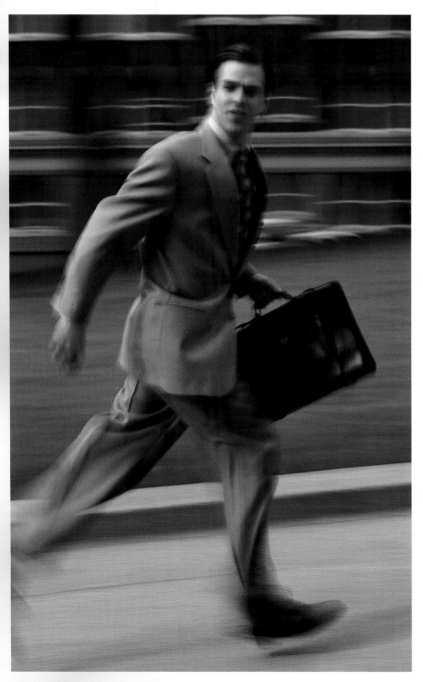

Below: Nux vomica people, highly-strung and impatient, are the entrepreneurs of society and thrive on challenge.

Phosphorous

Phosphorous types are great fun to be with, and they're kind and affectionate. But don't expect them to help in an emergency. Faced with a crisis they tend to go to pieces. Any form of stress or illness makes them indifferent to others, but they're apt to be demanding when they themselves need sympathy. When life is going well, they're usually in the best of health. If things go wrong, they're likely to suffer badly from tension. Other possible problems for this type include respiratory trouble, nausea, vomiting, constipation and neuralgia.

Pulsatilla

People of the Pulsatilla type, often women, are affectionate, gentle and almost too agreeable. They may appear to be doormats, walked over by employers, family and friends – but can exhibit a degree of stubbornness if pushed too far. They love children, animals, nature and fresh air. Most of their problems can be described as women's ailments. Other possible traumas include coughs and colds, eye infections and digestive troubles. If they feel off colour, they are apt to be weepy, but respond with enthusiasm to expressions of affection.

Below: Phosphorous types are great fun to be with, and they're kind and affectionate.

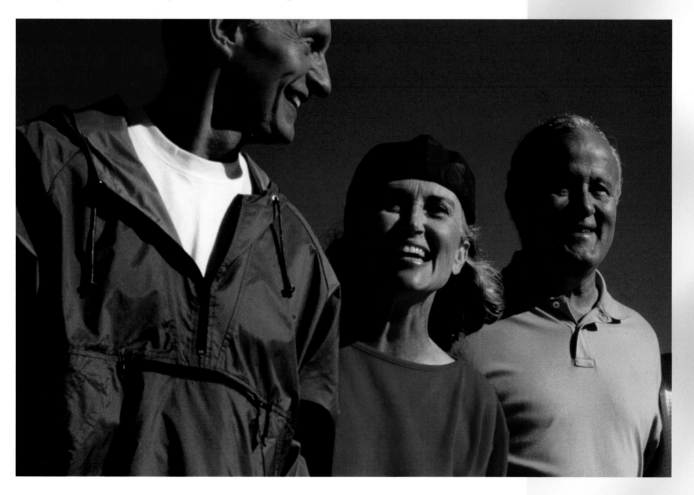

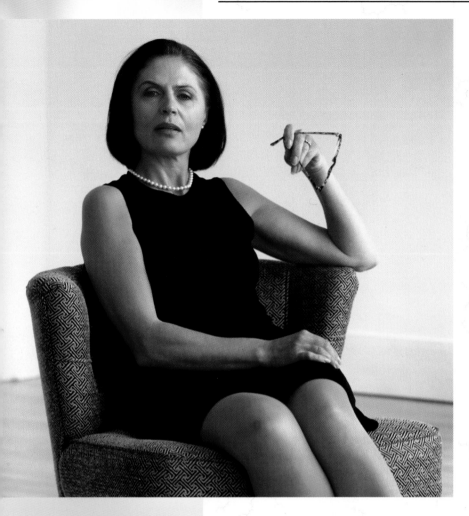

Above: Sepia people are usually extremely elegant and, on social occasions, seem extrovert and self-possessed.

Silica

People of this type are not very strong. Usually thin and pale, they frequently suffer from colds. Despite their lack of mental and physical stamina, they are hard workers, often to the extent that exhaustion results. They find it difficult to reach decisions and have no confidence in their own abilities, yet they can be stubborn. Silica types can suffer from a variety of fairly minor problems. These include poor condition of the skin, teeth, hair and nails, recurrent colds, ear infections, headaches, coughs and a weak digestive system.

Sulphur

Intellectual, highly imaginative, inventive – and hopelessly untidy. This is the typical Sulphur type. These people are full of bright ideas, but lack the practical skills or organisation to put them into practice. They are totally self-centred, yet generous and good-humoured, so that friends tend to overlook their myriad faults. They suffer mainly from disorders of the digestion and the skin, but other problems may include menopausal problems in women and impotence in men.

Sepia

Sepia people are usually extremely elegant and, on social occasions, seem extrovert and self-possessed. However, this veneer disappears when they are alone with their family. They can be irritable and reluctant to accept any responsibility. Extreme fatigue can be troublesome. They tire quickly and weep easily, but reject sympathy and will go to great lengths to conceal their vulnerability. Typically, Sepia is linked with women's problems – ailments of the ovaries, vagina and uterus and a lack of interest in sex.

IT'S UP TO YOU

Keeping a record

You are much more likely to gain significant results from homeopathic treatment if you give the practitioner your whole-hearted co-operation. Indeed, some practitioners ask their patients to keep a detailed written record of every manifestation of their symptoms and their own reactions to them.

It is not enough to note merely "headache better" or "inner discomfort". The symptoms that most concern your homeopath are those that have meaning to you. These are the very symptoms that will guide them in prescribing a remedy. You should make a note, too, if you feel that there could be a reason for the headache lessening or for the inner discomfort. The headache may be less troublesome because you have increased your fluid intake or because you have been able to spend more time in the fresh air. Perhaps the inner discomfort was caused by over-indulgence at a business lunch. Write down whatever you think is the reason for your condition.

In the beginning, you will find it difficult to decide just how detailed your reports should be. Don't worry about that. Just be careful not to invent symptoms and reactions merely so that you have something to report. At the same time, don't try to rationalise your feelings, for fear of seeming self-centred.

In a nutshell, your practitioner would like you to tell them about every deviation from the norm – on all levels. This includes your mental and emotional reactions as well as the physical ones.

Below: in the beginning, you will find it difficult to decide just how detailed your reports to your homeopath should be.

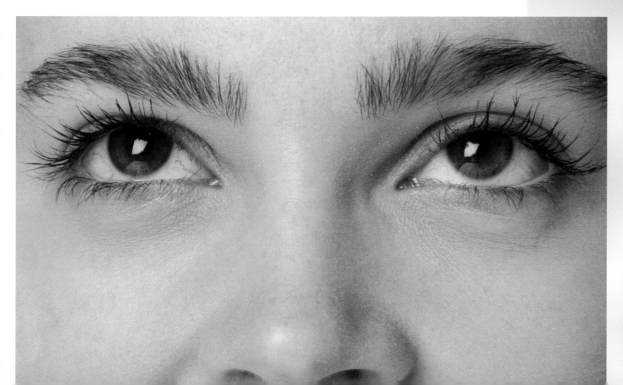

Changing your lifestyle

Homeopathy is thought to stimulate the body's powers of self-healing, but you can do a lot to assist the process. There is little point in your practitioner carefully prescribing a remedy that is exactly right for you if you spend most of your time slouched in front of the television set, smoking and eating fast food. It is up to you to decide, here and now, that you will do everything in your power to ensure your return to good health. And having made that decision – do it!

Below: you can do a lot to aid the healing process by eating sensibly.

In this health-conscious age, there cannot be many people who are unaware of how to maintain a reasonable standard of well-being. Nobody is asking you to become a health freak. However, there are a few well-tried methods to help you keep in good shape – in every sense of the words.

Eating and drinking

Obviously, you need to eat sensibly. That doesn't mean you must exist on raw vegetables, sunflower seeds and water. It does mean that you should follow a few simple rules.

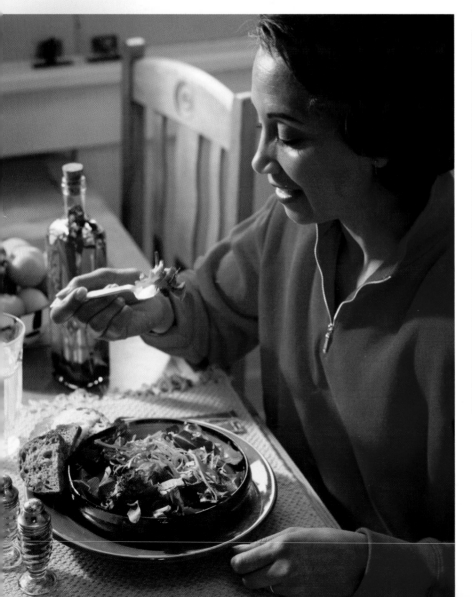

> *Drink plenty of fluids – water, fruit juice, etc. – and reduce the amount of coffee and tea you consume. Some homeopaths will advise you to cut out caffeine-loaded drinks completely.*
>
> *Eat fish and poultry rather than red meat.*
>
> *Restrict your intake of processed foods, fats, salt and sugar.*
>
> *Eat as much salad, fruit and vegetables as you wish.*
>
> *Once you get used to these simple rules, you'll find that a healthy diet doesn't hurt a bit!*

Keep moving

It's important not to be a couch potato but, then again, you are not expected to run a marathon or spend every night at the gym. The best way to get moving is to put a little more effort into everything you do.

Run up the stairs, instead of plodding. Walk briskly to the shops, swinging your arms and smiling. Shove the vacuum cleaner around energetically. When you hear music on the radio, prance around the room and dance to it.

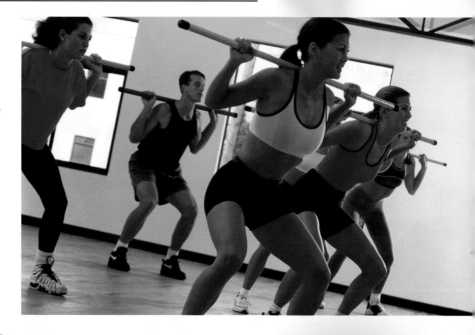

Take a brisk walk in the open air every day, even when it's raining.

Make a conscious effort to deepen your breathing.

Join an exercise class – they're available for every age group and a great way to meet people.

Swim as often as possible – and if you can't swim, learn how.

And, in general…

Ensure you get sufficient sleep.

Consider taking up meditation. It's incredibly relaxing.

Find an absorbing interest, pastime or recreation.

Try to adopt a positive attitude.

Don't …

Smoke.

Drink to excess.

Worry.

Forget to SMILE.

Suggestions, not rules

All the ideas listed here are merely suggestions that will help you to gain the most from your homeopathic treatment. You're not expected to make any drastic changes in your lifestyle – though some people do, and love the result. All you are required to do is accept the responsibility for your own well-being. Adopt these habits – or some of them. Co-operate with your homeopath and you'll never look back.

Above: join an exercise class – they're available for every age group and a great way to meet people.

D.I.Y. HOMEOPATHY

Undoubtedly, homeopathic self-treatment is a viable option for a number of minor common ailments.

As we have already seen, most homeopathic remedies can be bought over the counter at health shops and pharmacies. Theoretically, therefore, it should be a simple matter to obtain the medicines you want.

Below: most homeopathic remedies can be bought over the counter at health shops and pharmacies.

Bear in mind, though, that when you visit a homeopathic practitioner the remedy he prescribes will be suited to your individual requirements, taking into account every aspect of you, your personality, lifestyle, etc. Over-the-counter remedies cannot possibly be so specific. That being so, it is vital that you should make every attempt to select those most likely to alleviate the condition from which you are suffering.

DIAGNOSIS

Obviously, your first concern must be to diagnose your ailment. You will need to make a list of the symptoms from which you are suffering.

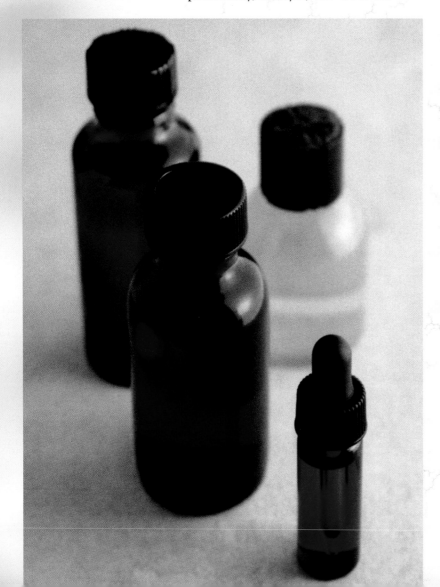

Identify the worst symptoms and then consider others less severe.

Can you suggest what may have caused these symptoms?

Where do they occur, how often do they happen and how distressing are they?

Are these symptoms affected, for better or worse, by any particular condition or situation?

Are you suffering from any psychological problems that could cause or affect the symptoms?

CONSULT THE EXPERTS

Your next step should be to look up your symptoms in one of the many homeopathic guides available. This will enable you to compare your symptoms with the various remedies listed. This may be difficult, because certain symptoms are common to a wide variety of ailments.

For example, a sore throat may indicate tonsillitis, incipient influenza – or simply that you spent too long talking in a smoky pub last night. Diarrhoea usually suggests food poisoning, but it can be caused by excessive worry or even IBS (irritable bowel syndrome.) Or, of course, perhaps you had one drink too many. Any good homeopathic directory will suggest suitable remedies for these and other common ailments, but it is up to you to decide exactly which symptoms you are exhibiting and, therefore, which remedy you should use.

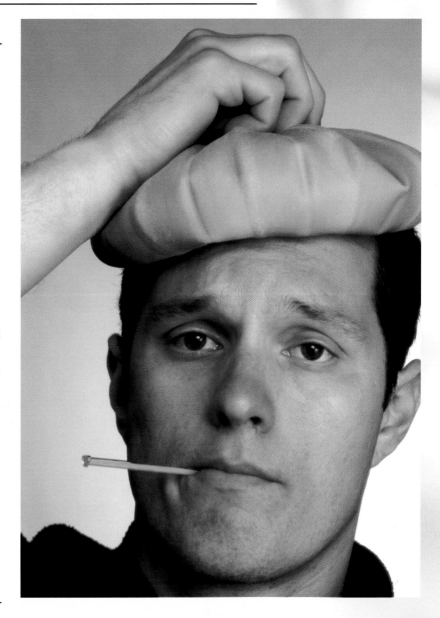

TYPES OF REMEDY

There are two kinds of homeopathic remedy. The first is the classic type, which contains only one ingredient. Thus, if you buy Nux vomica to alleviate an attack of hiccups, Nux vomica will be the only constituent.

The second type is known as the indicated remedy, which means that it is a combination of ingredients suitable for treating any one ailment. It may contain up to three ingredients.

Homeopathic medicines can be obtained as tinctures and ointments, in powder form or granules. More usually, they are found in the form of lactose tablets, which should be dissolved under the tongue.

Above: look up your symptoms in one of the many homeopathic guides available and compare them with the various remedies listed.

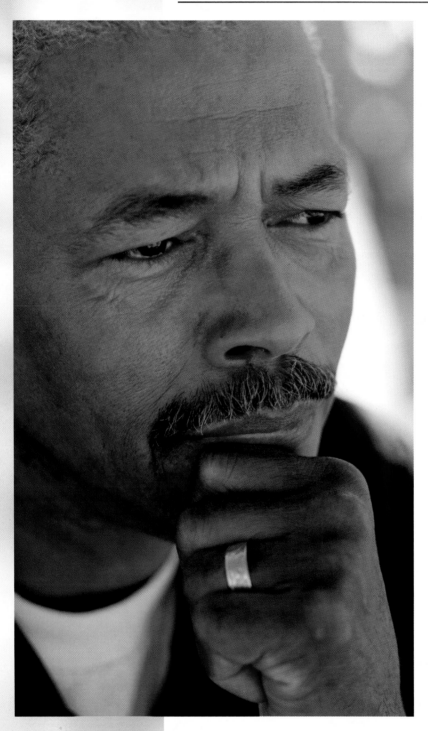

Above: the initial reaction will probably be psychological.

one problem at a time. For example, if you take Belladonna to alleviate severe earache, resist the temptation to also dose yourself with Ipecacuanha for bronchitis. By treating only one disorder and taking only one remedy at a time, you should know within a few hours whether or not it works for you. If it doesn't, you may then select another remedy to try. And, if that doesn't work either, wait another few hours and try a third.

REACTIONS

Fairly soon after taking the remedy you will know if you have chosen the right one. The initial reaction will probably be psychological. Suddenly you will begin to feel more cheerful and optimistic. Hopefully, you will notice an improvement in your physical condition a short time later.

If the symptoms don't improve or if they worsen, then you have probably chosen the wrong remedy. Don't worry. This cannot harm you. Stop taking it and check again with your reference book to find something more appropriate to your symptoms. You will find that minor chronic conditions take longer to respond to a remedy. Acute problems are often quickly solved.

ONE AT A TIME

If this is your first venture into the field of homeopathic self-treatment, you are strongly advised to treat only

SIDE-EFFECTS

When you begin homeopathic treatment, you may find that your symptoms are intensified. This is what Dr Hahnemann called an "aggravation". It occurs because the remedy has boosted your immune system, which is fighting the illness. This type of side-effect indicates that you have selected the right remedy. It's as well to stop taking the tablets until the reaction subsides, then resume treatment.

SAFETY MEASURES

If you are receiving medication from your GP, you should not stop taking it until you have discussed the situation with him.

Similarly, if you are pregnant or breast-feeding, you should consult your GP or practitioner before taking homeopathic remedies.

DON'T RUSH

With homeopathy, it's very much a case of "softly, softly, catchee monkey". Don't be tempted to rush into prescribing for yourself until you have carefully checked symptoms against remedies. Prescribing the wrong remedy will not harm you, but your condition could worsen because of the delay in identifying the right one. As you gain more experience, your confidence and your diagnostic expertise will increase. If, at any time, your condition fails to improve, you are strongly advised to seek the help of a qualified practitioner.

Below: don't be tempted to rush into prescribing for yourself until you have carefully checked symptoms against remedies.

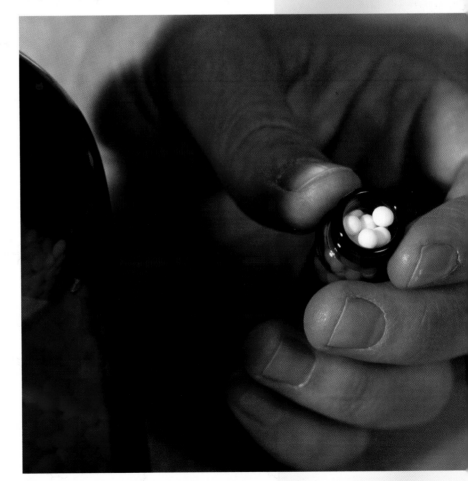

Below: a health-conscious lifestyle – a balanced diet, plenty of sleep, fresh air and exercise – supports homeopathic remedies.

Far right: proper functioning of the heart is essential to life and any problem with the circulatory system should be regarded seriously.

SUPPORTING THE REMEDY

Homeopathy is an holistic therapy. The remedies are designed to promote the body's self-healing powers but you, the patient, can do a lot to support the action of the medicine you have chosen. All homeopathic treatment will work better if it is combined with a health-conscious lifestyle – a balanced diet, plenty of sleep, fresh air and exercise.

Remember, too, that you should not eat, drink or brush your teeth for 30 minutes before or after taking a homeopathic remedy. Steer clear, too, of strong flavours and spicy foods

And finally – it is important that you should not handle the medicine. Tip the dose from the bottle on to a clean dry spoon and thence into your mouth.

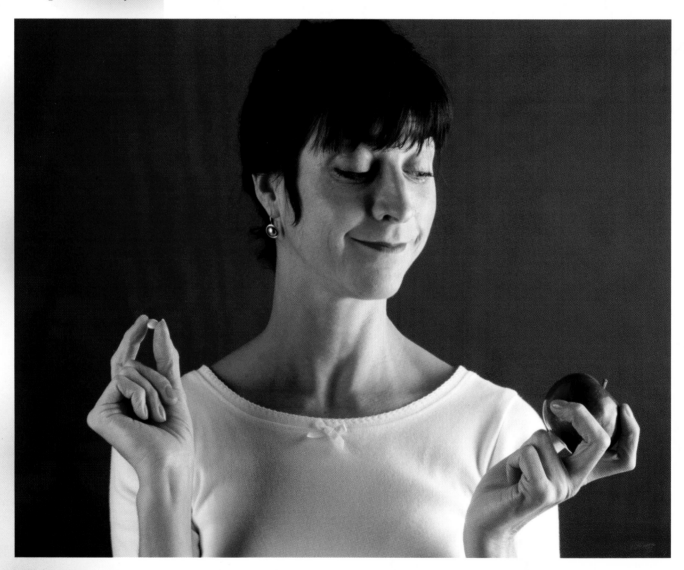

DON'T TAKE IT FOR GRANTED

We all tend to take good health for granted – until something goes wrong. Then, all too often, we realise how little we know about that extremely intricate machine, the human body.

This section of the book gives a brief outline of the various systems of your body, names a few of the minor ailments to which they are most susceptible and suggests homeopathic remedies that may help.

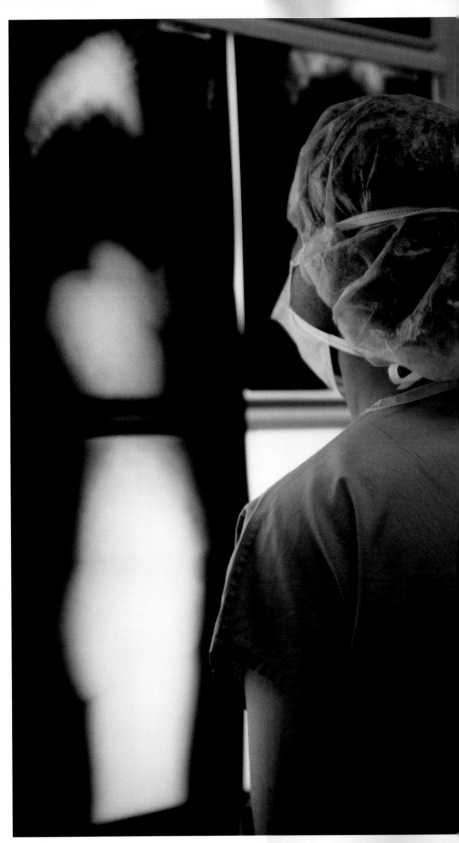

THE CIRCULATORY SYSTEM

The job of the heart and blood vessels is to maintain a constant flow of blood throughout the body. Also known as the cardiovascular system, the circulatory system supplies body tissues with essential oxygen and other nutrients. It also carries away waste products.

Proper functioning of the heart is essential to life and any problem with the circulatory system should be regarded seriously.

COMMON PROBLEMS

ANGINA PECTORIS

Angina is characterised by a severe cramping pain in the middle of the chest. It sometimes spreads to the neck and jaw and down the left arm.

Causes
Angina is an indication that insufficient oxygen is reaching the heart, usually because of narrowing of the arteries. An attack can be brought on by shock, over-exertion, intense cold, or over-eating.

Symptoms include chest pain, nausea, dizziness and sweating.

What to do
Rest and relax. Even if the pain eases up fairly quickly, don't rush into action at once. If you are a smoker, throw away your cigarettes and resolve never to light one again.

Help!
Chest pain should always be treated seriously, particularly in the elderly, diabetics and smokers. The first attack of angina can be very frightening and you are advised to consult a doctor as soon as possible, if only for reassurance. They will almost certainly advise you to watch your weight and to start a programme of gentle exercise.

> ### REMEDIES
>
> *Violent pain and numbness in fingers* – **Latrodectus**
>
> *Faintness, breathing difficulties* – **Naja**
>
> *Chest feels constricted, breathing problems* – **Cactus**
>
> NB: *These remedies are suitable for mild or infrequent attacks of angina. Constitutional homeopathic treatment may be needed (see page 28), depending on the cause of the condition and how often it recurs.*

Below: angina is charac-terised by a severe cramping pain in the middle of the chest.

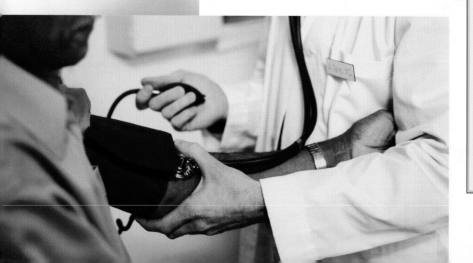

VARICOSE VEINS AND HAEMORRHOIDS

Varicose veins usually occur in the legs, but can also be found in the rectum and the anus (as haemorrhoids). The tendency to this problem is often inherited and is four times more common in women than in men.

Causes

If you spend a lot of time standing or if you are overweight, you are likely to suffer from varicose veins. Contributory factors also include a sedentary lifestyle, the menopause and advancing age. Haemorrhoids are often the result of constipation.

What to do

Support tights help to reduce the discomfort of varicose veins. Never stand if you can sit and if you can put your feet up – do so. Sit and sleep with your feet raised slightly above the level of the hips. Regular gentle exercise is also helpful.

Avoid constipation by increasing your intake of fruit and vegetables and by drinking plenty of water.

Help!

Seek medical help if the condition worsens or is persistent. This is particularly important if bleeding is caused, either by a blow or because the vein has burst.

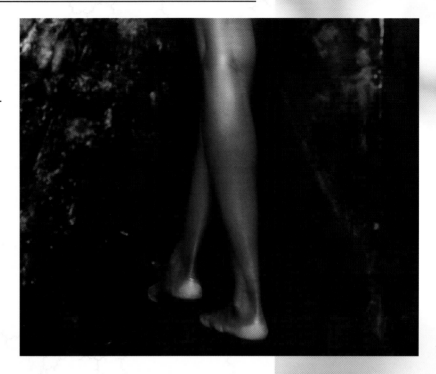

Consult your doctor if you suffer from constipation for more than a few days. If bleeding from the anus occurs, do not assume that haemorrhoids cause it. See the doctor immediately.

Above: varicose veins usually occur in the legs,

REMEDIES

Skin is mottled and discoloured
– **Carbo veg.**

Veins feel sore and bruised
– **Hamamelis**

Haemorrhoids

Itching and burning pain
– **Paeonia ointment**

Anus feeling sore and bruised
– **Hamamelis**

Anaemia

There are several types of anaemia, but some symptoms are common to them all. These include pallor, fainting, palpitations, fatigue, headaches and breathlessness.

Causes

Anaemia is usually caused by a deficiency of iron. It can also occur because of blood loss following an accident or surgery, heavy menstruation, or peptic ulcers.

What to do

If you notice any of the above named symptoms, increase your intake of green vegetables and salad. Consult your doctor if the symptoms worsen or last for longer than a couple of weeks.

Help!

Your doctor will almost certainly arrange for you to have blood tests. They may also prescribe an iron supplement.

NB: It is unwise to take supplements for anaemia until you have received medical advice.

Below: your doctor will almost certainly arrange for you to have blood tests. They may also prescribe an iron supplement.

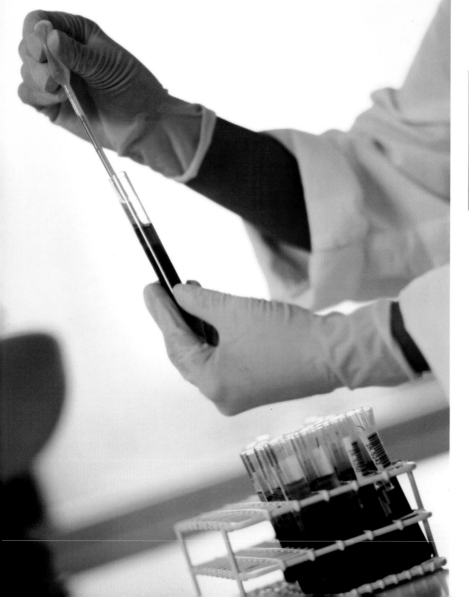

Remedies

Homeopathic treatment will depend on your constitutional type (see page 28), but a diet rich in iron and Vitamin B12 may also be prescribed.

THE DIGESTIVE SYSTEM

As already explained, the digestive system begins with the breaking down of food in the mouth. It ends when waste products are expelled from the rectum. A healthy digestion goes a long way towards maintaining general good health. However, in these days of fast food, too many people consume an inferior diet and rely on antacids to relieve the consequent discomfort.

COMMON PROBLEMS

INDIGESTION AND HEARTBURN

Any discomfort in the chest or upper abdomen is usually described as indigestion. Symptoms may include flatulence, heartburn, wind, hiccups or nausea. Quite severe pain can also be present.

Heartburn, said to regularly afflict 25% of British adults, causes a burning acidic discomfort in the chest.

Causes
There are many reasons for the onset of indigestion and heartburn. These include eating too much too quickly, swallowing air, pregnancy, stress, or being overweight.

What to do
Eat slowly and rest for half an hour on conclusion of a meal. Don't eat between meals. Avoid foods that you know you find difficult to digest. Follow a diet rich in fibre. Avoid over-the-counter indigestion remedies. If taken to excess, they can often cause the condition to worsen.

Help!
If pain persists for more than four or five hours, if you suffer from prolonged vomiting or if you vomit blood, seek medical advice immediately. This is particularly important should the vomit resemble coffee grounds.

REMEDIES

Excessive flatulence. Pain when eating
– **Carbo veg.**

Pain with nausea/vomiting
– **Pulsatilla**

Heartburn

Acid discomfort, constant hunger
– **Phosphorous**

Desire for sweet, fatty foods
– **Sulphur**

Far right: abdominal griping spasms and irregular bowel habits.

IRRITABLE BOWEL SYNDROME

IBS is typified by abdominal griping spasms and irregular bowel habits. This can result in diarrhoea and/or constipation, a swollen abdomen and the feeling that evacuation is incomplete. It is believed that as many as 13% of British people – many of them middle-aged women – regularly experience these problems.

Causes
Precise causes for the onset of IBS are difficult to pinpoint.
Severe stress can produce an attack "out of the blue". Other possible causes are low-fibre diet or food allergies, such as intolerance of wheat or dairy products.

Below: other possible causes of IBS are low-fibre diet or food allergies, such as intolerance of wheat or dairy products.

What to do
It is important to remain as calm as possible if you develop IBS. Worry and stress will only aggravate the problem. Boost your fluid intake, but steer clear of alcohol. Try to decide which foods may intensify the symptoms. To do this, remove one particular item from the diet for four or five days. When reintroduced, take note of the symptoms. Are they still present or have they stopped?

Help!
If your bowel habits have recently changed or if blood appears in the stools, consult a doctor. Similarly, if diarrhoea is so severe that you are afraid to go out, seek medical advice. Your doctor may prescribe bulking agents.

If IBS comes on suddenly, it is worth consulting your doctor about it in order to rule out more serious ailments.

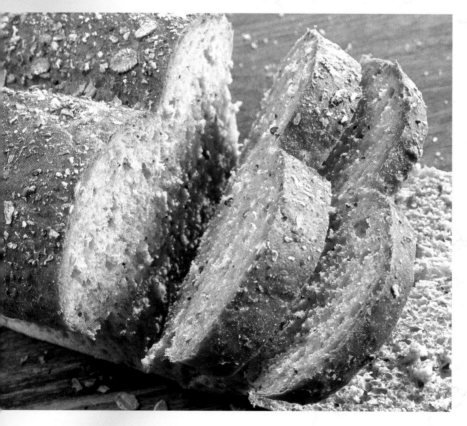

REMEDIES

Alternating constipation/diarrhoea
– **Argent. nit.**

Flatulence and griping spasms
– **Nux vomica**

Severe diarrhoea and colic
– **Arsen. alb.**

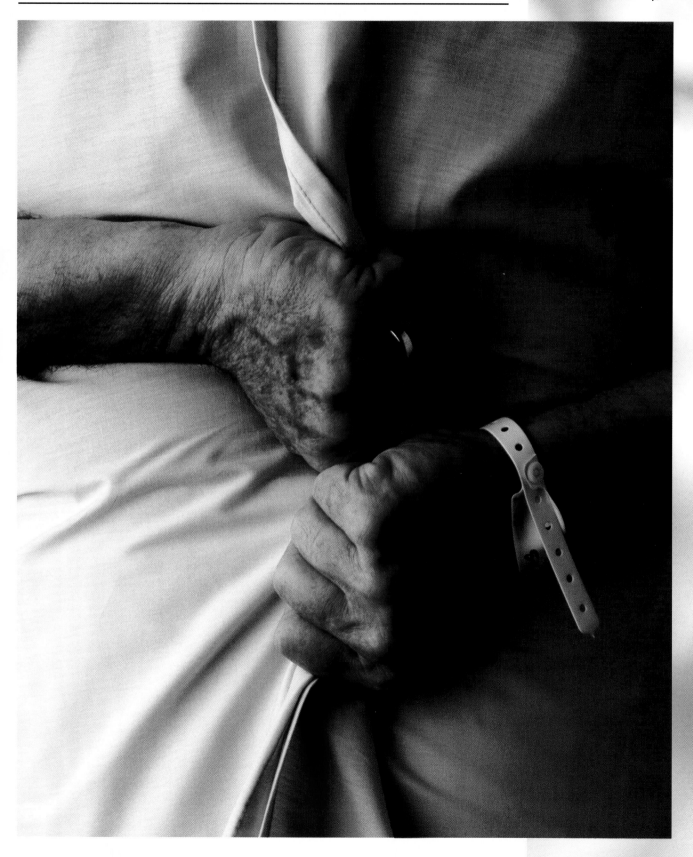

MUSCULO-SKELETAL SYSTEM

The function of the musculo-skeletal system is to protect the internal organs of the body and to give it mobility.

The most common problem related to this system is damage related to wear and tear. This is often the case with elderly people, because of the thinning of the bones. Such damage may take a long time to heal. In younger people, problems may be caused by injuries, but these usually respond swiftly to treatment.

Below: the most common problem related to this system is damage related to wear and tear, sometimes due to ageing.

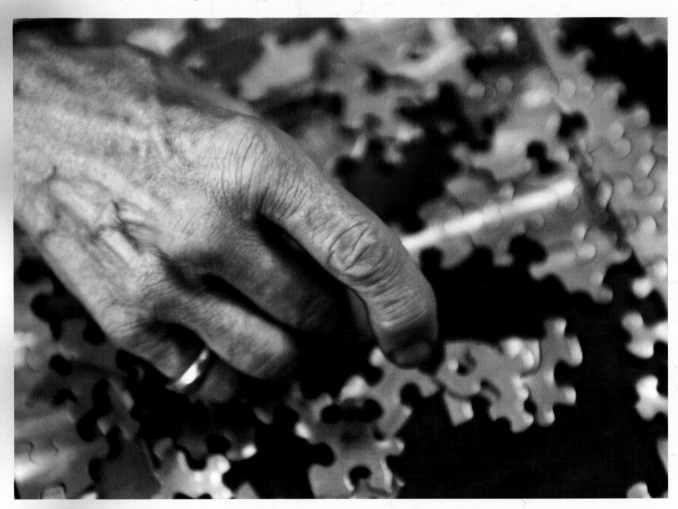

COMMON PROBLEMS

OSTEOARTHRITIS

This is a degenerative disease, almost synonymous with old age. X-rays of elderly people show that up to 85% of them have some signs of osteoarthritis, even if they have no symptoms.

Symptoms include stiffness and pain in the joints, swelling, inflammation and, in some cases, deformity.

Causes
Some forms of osteoarthritis can be hereditary and it tends to afflict more women than men. In other cases, inflammation and pain can occur on the site of a long-forgotten injury.

What to do
It is wise to consult a doctor immediately you feel any pain or stiffness in a joint. Rest as much as possible and apply warmth to the affected joint, but try to keep it moving gently. Walking, cycling or swimming can help.

Help!
Your doctor will probably prescribe painkillers and/or anti-inflammatory drugs. He will certainly advise you to lose any excess weight. In severe cases, surgical intervention may be necessary in the form of a joint replacement.

REMEDIES

Pain and stiffness on waking
– Rhus tox.

Joints painful, swollen and hot
– Bryonia

Inflammation and production of fluid
– Apis

Consultation with a professional homeopath is advised as much can be done to alleviate the severe pain associated with this illness. Constitutional remedies include Kali. carb., Lycopodium, Nat. mur., Pulsatilla and Sulphur.

Below: walking, cycling or swimming can help ease the symptoms of osteoarthritis

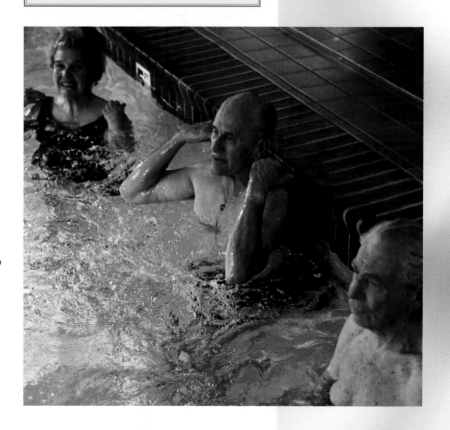

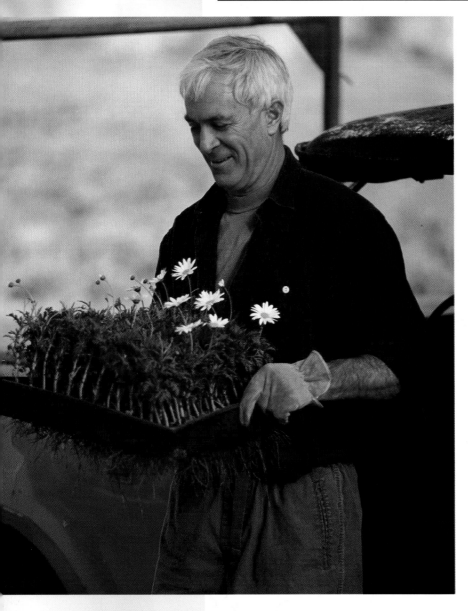

the result of lifting something heavy if you are unused to such tasks. Sleeping in an awkward position can be to blame. There are dozens of explanations for backache and it is often impossible to pinpoint the cause.

What to do
The traditional remedy for backache is resting on a hard bed (with a board pushed beneath the mattress) or on the floor. A hot water bottle applied to the back may ease the pain, as may mild analgesics. Backache will be worsened if you are overweight.

Help!
Severe prolonged back pain merits medical attention, but most doctors freely admit that diagnosis is difficult. Your GP may prescribe painkillers and, if the condition is serious, may send you for X-ray. They may recommend physiotherapy or suggest you consult a chiropractor.

Above: people most likely to suffer from back pain are those with heavy lifting jobs.

BACKACHE

At least 75% of all adults suffer from backache at one time or another and it is the primary cause for time off work for illness.

Causes
People most likely to suffer from back pain are those with heavy lifting jobs. However, it can also occur as

REMEDIES

Pain in the small of the back – **Kali. carb.**

Soreness down the spine. – *Kali. phos.*

Stiffness and pain in lower back and neck – **Ferrum met.**

Lower back pain radiating down thigh – **Berberis**

CRAMP

The agonising pain of cramp occurs when muscles go into spasm, and is the result of a shortage of oxygen or a build-up of lactic acid. The pain usually lasts for only a matter of seconds, but can be more prolonged.

Causes

Cramp often occurs during or immediately after exercise and athletes are particularly prone to suffer in this way. Other causes include sitting or lying in an awkward position, or any excessive repetitive movement – i.e. writer's cramp. Night cramps are common, but usually have no known cause.

What to do

Stretching or firm massage of the muscles involved may bring some relief. If you suffer from leg cramps during the night, it may help if you raise the foot of your bed by about four inches (10cm).

Help!

See your GP if you frequently suffer from severe cramp. They may refer you to a consultant or suggest an EMG (electromyogram) examination.

REMEDIES

Severe cramp in feet or legs
– Cuprum met.

Cramp after prolonged exercise
– Arnica

NB: Consult a doctor at once if you suffer cramp in your chest during or after exercise.

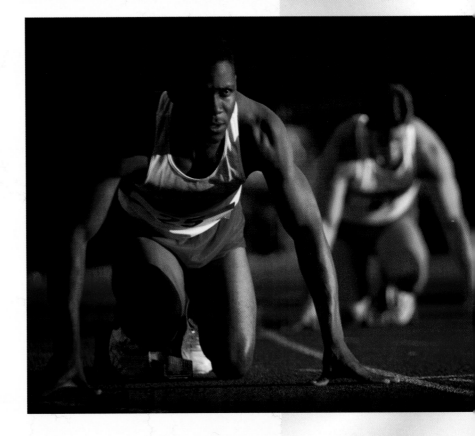

Below: cramp often occurs during or immediately after exercise and athletes are particularly prone to suffer in this way.

THE NERVOUS SYSTEM

The body's computer

Your nervous system is similar to a powerful computer designed to control an extremely complex machine.

The 14 billion nerve cells in the brain are particularly vulnerable to damage and lack the ability to repair themselves. Obviously, therefore, serious problems – such as a stroke – require immediate consultation with a medical doctor. On the other hand, a number of everyday ailments respond swiftly to homeopathic treatment.

COMMON PROBLEMS

HEADACHES

Even if you have suffered from headaches for years, you may find that homeopathic treatment produces a common response. However, you should carefully consider the root cause of the pain, as a constant headache can be a warning of a serious illness.

Below: some people are more likely than others to suffer from headaches.

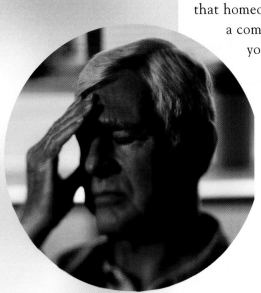

Causes

Some people are more likely than others to suffer from headaches. This has much to do with the sufferer's constitutional type (see page 28). Causes can include stress, fatigue, eyestrain, over-eating or hunger, over-indulgence in alcohol – or something as simple as dozing in an uncomfortable position.

What to do

If the headache results from over-indulgence in food or drink, a dose of Alka-Seltzer is probably the best remedy. If it is caused by stress or over-work, a walk in the fresh air and/or a sound sleep is indicated. Drink plenty of water. You can try homeopathic remedies (see below), but if no relief is obtained, see a doctor.

Help!

Medical consultation is imperative if the headache follows a head injury, if your temperature is higher than 38ªC, if there is nausea and vomiting or if the pain lasts for more than a couple of days.

REMEDIES

For sudden onset headaches
– **Aconite**

For "hangover" headaches
– **Nux vomica**

MIGRAINE

Anyone who classifies migraine as "a sort of headache" is obviously not a sufferer. Migraine has been described as the worst headache in the world. Symptoms include nausea, vomiting and visual disturbances, in addition to severe pain, usually on one side of the head.

Causes

If you are a martyr to migraine, you will probably already know what causes your problems. Migraine has many "triggers", which vary widely from person to person. So far as food is concerned, peanuts, chocolate, oranges, cheese and red wine are common culprits. A missed meal may also provoke an attack.

Other causes include fatigue, flashing lights, noise, excessive heat and excitement, even of the pleasurable kind.

What to do

If you are a migraine sufferer, you will probably notice warning signs (i.e. visual disturbances) before the onset of the full-blown attack. A cup of tea and some dry toast may help to nip it in the bud.

If you have never suffered from migraine before or if the attack descends without warning, the only remedy is to rest in a darkened room. Some people find relief from placing a cold damp face flannel on the forehead, others prefer to rest the head on a covered hot water bottle. Most sufferers eventually discover for themselves what best alleviates this miserable condition.

Help!

Because symptoms of migraine can be so severe, it is sometimes difficult to decide when to seek medical help. For this reason, too, it is sensible to keep in your first aid kit the remedies listed below. You should also follow the advice given for "ordinary" headaches.

Should you have any reason to feel that the symptoms are especially extreme, do not hesitate to phone a doctor and ask for advice. You will find that most medical professionals, far from regarding migraine as a trivial problem, are quick to respond to this type of situation.

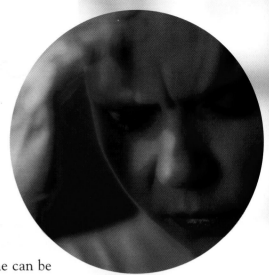

Above: migraine has been described as the worst headache in the world.

REMEDIES

Pain mainly on right side of the head – **Lycopodium**

Severe pain causing tearfulness – **Pulsatilla**

Blinding pain on top of head with tingling in the lips and tongue – **Nat. mur.**

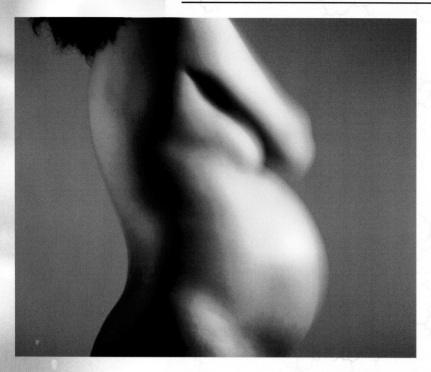

Above: Sciatica is usually caused by pressure on the nerve and is particularly common in pregnant women.

SCIATICA

The pain of sciatica usually affects the buttock and thigh, on one side, but it sometimes extends right down the leg. Numbness and weakness may also occur and, in severe cases, the pain may extend to both legs.

Causes
Sciatica is usually caused by pressure on the nerve and is particularly common in pregnant women. It can also result from muscle spasm or simply from sleeping in an awkward position. The reason for sciatic pain is often difficult to pinpoint, since any neurological disorder can produce it.

What to do
Placing a covered hot water bottle on the affected area may give temporary relief. Ensure that your bed has a fairly firm mattress. Resting flat on your back may help to relieve the pain. Conversely, gentle movement can have a beneficial effect.

Help!
It is seldom necessary to seek emergency treatment for sciatica. Despite the pain it causes, it is not a dangerous ailment. Nonetheless, if the pain is of long standing or worsens, it is advisable to take medical advice, if only to eradicate the complications previously mentioned.

REMEDIES

Sciatic pain worsens when sitting – **Ammonium mur.**

Pain worsens in cold, damp weather – **Colocynthis**

Pain is relieved by movement and warmth – **Rhus tox.**

Dealing with disorders of the nervous system
Homeopathy's holistic approach is particularly useful when dealing with any problems connected with the nervous system. The suggested remedies are especially helpful during recuperation. They will then calm any agitation produced by pain and thereby stimulate the body's natural healing tendencies.

THE EARS

Apart from washing your ears, you probably don't pay much attention to them. Yet, in addition to interpreting the sound waves that are around us 24 hours a day, these intricate sensory organs are also responsible for maintaining our balance.

Ears are susceptible to a wide variety of disorders and easily damaged. Invasion by micro-organisms or minute specks of any foreign body may cause vertigo (disturbance of the inner ear) or other serious problems that could lead to deafness.

Any discomfort or pain associated with the ear requires immediate professional investigation. If you feel that your ear is blocked or that there is some foreign object inside it, consult your doctor. On no account should you probe inside the ear or attempt to wash it out with water.

Below: any discomfort or pain associated with the ear requires immediate professional investigation.

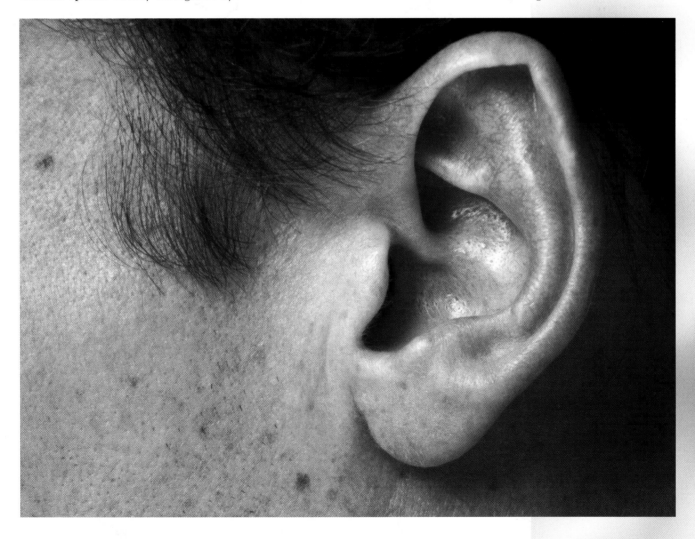

COMMON PROBLEMS

TINNITUS

Because tinnitus is not a visible complaint, sufferers often feel that other people lack sympathy for the problems it causes. The noise of tinnitus varies, but can be extremely stressful. It can be persistent or intermittent – a high-pitched whistle, a rushing roaring sound, or anything in between.

Causes
Tinnitus may be a result of ageing or of working in a noisy environment. It can also be caused by influenza or by a reaction to certain drugs such as quinine and aspirin. It may result from a head injury, from flying or simply excess wax in the ear.

What to do
One of the worst aspects of tinnitus is the tension and stress it causes. Try some relaxation techniques to combat this. If you have neck problems of any description, consult a chiropractitioner or physio-therapist.

Help!
It is unlikely that tinnitus will ever cause any sort of crisis or emergency. However, you would be well advised to consult a doctor as soon as the condition appears. Too many people tend to shrug off the onset of ear noise as an inescapable part of ageing. This is not necessarily so, and it is always advisable to ask for help.

Below: the noise of tinnitus varies, but can be extremely stressful.

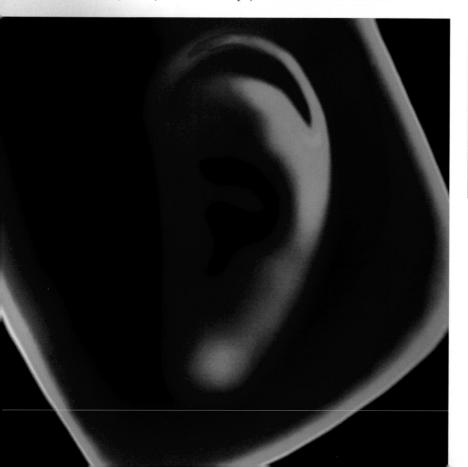

REMEDIES

Hissing sound. Ears feel blocked – **Carbon sulph.**

Buzzing in ears. Dizziness, sometimes with severe headache – **China sulph.**

EARACHE

Earache is a very common symptom with a variety of fairly minor causes. Nonetheless, it can cause severe pain and, should it continue, medical advice is needed.

Causes
One of the most common reasons for earache is a build-up of wax in the ear. Water in the ears, often caused by swimming, can also be to blame, and may lead to infection of the middle ear. A boil or an abscess, with the consequent build-up of pus, can cause intense pain.

What to do
Applying warmth to the ear, in the form of a covered hot water bottle, often alleviates the pain.

Help!
Professional help is needed if there is any discharge from the ear or if you begin to run a temperature. Any form of ear problem in a child should be referred to a doctor immediately.

REMEDIES

Acute throbbing pain – **Hepar. sulph.**

Intense pain with dry mouth and fever *–* **Belladonna**

Pain appears to be behind the ear drum – **Pulsatilla**

Dealing with ear problems
Although any persistent pain in the ear requires professional investigation, homeopathic remedies can be helpful. They are particularly useful in dealing with infection and work well if the pain is caused by catarrh resulting from a cough or cold.

Below: any form of ear problem in a child should be referred to a doctor immediately.

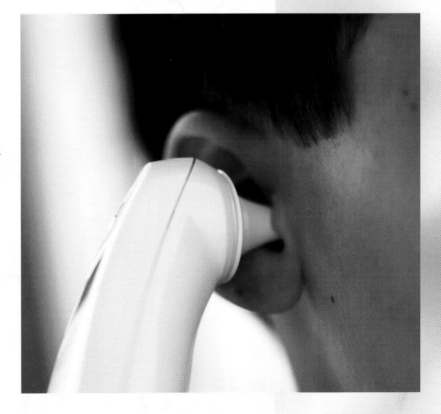

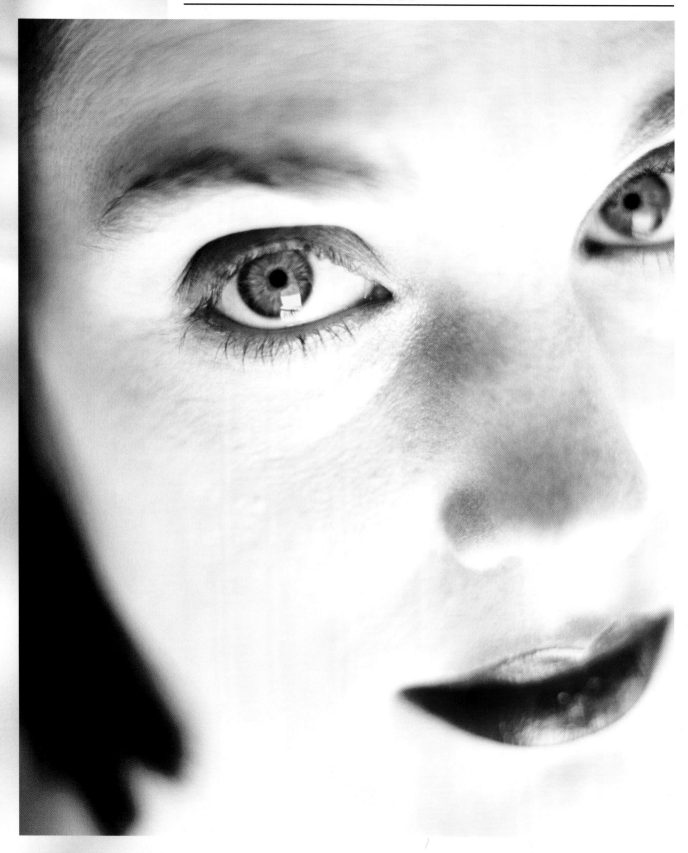

THE EYES

Your eyes are not only "the windows of your soul"; they are windows to the internal state of your body. A doctor can tell a great deal about the general state of your health by examining your eyes.

Irritation or infection of the eyes is common, due to the fact that they are constantly bombarded with pollutants – chemicals, dust, bacteria. Additionally, most of us rub our eyes much more frequently than we realise.

Eyestrain can produce a variety of discomforts, including migraine.

COMMON PROBLEMS

CONJUNCTIVITIS

Symptoms of conjunctivitis include inflammation, discomfort and a yellow discharge. This is a very common condition. It is estimated that one person in 50 gives conjunctivitis as the reason for visiting a doctor.

Causes

The problem is usually caused by infection, particularly in children. In adults, it can sometimes be the result of an allergy. Sharing a towel or frequently touching the eyes can spread infection. Changes in temperature can also worsen the situation, as can spending long periods in smoke-filled areas.

What to do

Bathe the eyes frequently. Remember always to sterilise the eye bath after each use. Rest the eyes as much as possible.

Help!

If the condition is severe, occurs frequently or lasts for more than a week, consult your doctor.

REMEDIES

For typical cases of conjunctivitis
*– **Euphrasia***

Far left: a doctor can tell a great deal about the general state of your health by examining your eyes.

Eyestrain

Eyestrain is typified by a sensation of tightness round the eyes, by blurring of the vision or by difficulty in changing the focus distance. A dull aching pain can be felt when moving the eyes and there is a "gritty" feeling to the lids.

Causes
Eyestrain is often caused by reading or working in a poor light. It can also be the result of over-work or stress.

What to do
Eyestrain can in some cases be completely avoided by frequent short breaks in concentration. Change the focus of your eyes and gaze into space for a few minutes. Place the palms of your hands over closed eyes and relax in the consequent darkness. Apply cold compresses to the eyes.

Help!
Persistent eyestrain merits a visit to your optician.

REMEDIES

Eyes sting and burn – **Ruta**

Eye movement is painful – **Nat. mur.**

Below: with eyestrain a dull aching pain can be felt when moving the eyes and there is a "gritty" feeling to the lids.

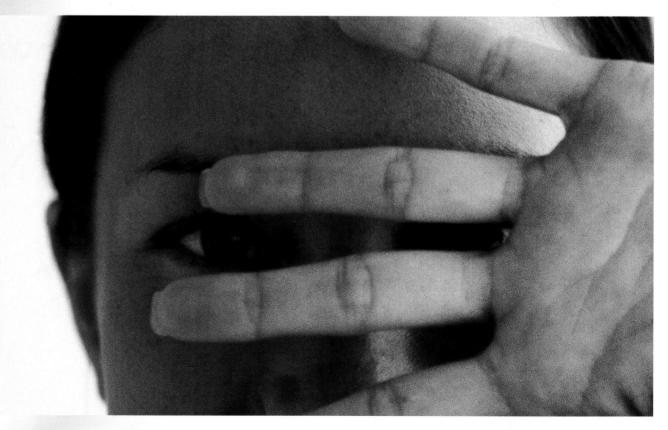

STYES

A stye is a small, pus-filled swelling at the base of the eyelashes. They are particularly common in children.

Causes
Infection is the most usual cause for the appearance of a stye. In children, a stye can result from frequent rubbing of the eyes when over-tired.

What to do
Use the eyes as little as possible. Operate a "hands off" policy, being particularly careful not to touch the "good" eye after you have touched the infected one. Bathing with hot boiled water may give some relief.

Help!
A stye will usually clear up within seven days and no medical help is necessary. If the condition recurs frequently, see your doctor in case you are run down.

REMEDIES

Eyes are swollen, inflamed and itchy – **Pulsatilla**

Eyes are red, swollen and painful – **Staphisagria**

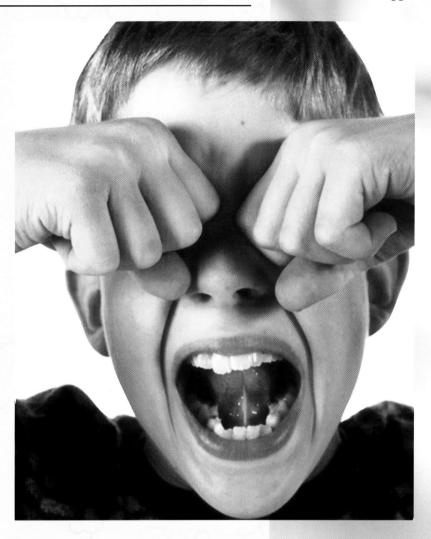

Dealing with eye problems
It is reassuring to know that relatively few eye disorders have anything to do with vision. In general, everyday eye problems are caused by infection, and homeopathy is particularly suited to dealing with this.

Nonetheless, long-standing or recurrent eye problems should be referred to a doctor or optician. Sight is much too valuable to risk.

Above: in children, a stye can result from frequent rubbing of the eyes when over-tired.

*Above: your general
health is shown by the
condition of the tongue
and the mucous
membranes of the mouth.*

*Far right: see a dentist as
soon as possible if you
experience swelling of
any kind – in the gums
or face or around the
tooth – or if you a
running a high
temperature.*

THE MOUTH

The mouth is the first part of the digestive system where the teeth break down food so that it can be swallowed. Your general health is shown by the condition of the tongue and the mucous membranes of the mouth.

The most common problems with the mouth are infections, dental problems and ulcers.

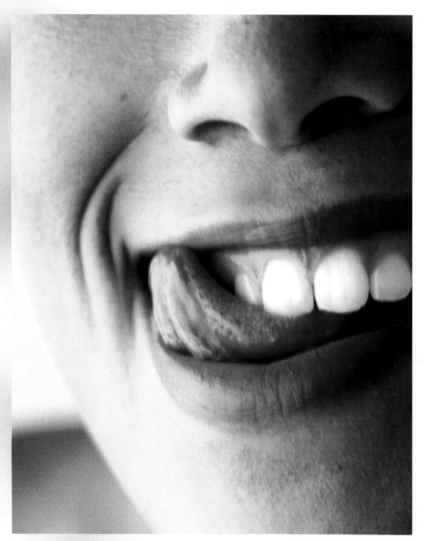

Common problems

MOUTH ULCERS

These are open sores or spots – white, grey or yellow – that occur inside the mouth, on the gums, lips or tongue.

Causes
These painful eruptions can occur if you are run-down or stressed. Other causes can be careless brushing of teeth or badly fitting dentures. Some women develop ulcers during their menstrual cycle. Mouth ulcers may also be indicative of a poor diet, food allergies, infection, stress or exhaustion.

What to do
Pay strict attention to mouth hygiene. Avoid spicy foods. Stop smoking. Use a saline mouthwash several times daily.

Help!
If the ulcers persist for more than a couple of weeks, consult your doctor. They may recommend antiseptic lozenges or analgesics to relieve the pain.

REMEDIES

---

*Ulcers with burning sensation
– **Arsen. alb.***

TOOTHACHE

This is usually an indication of tooth decay and can be extremely painful.

Causes

The most common cause of toothache is erosion of tooth enamel, exposing the inner part of the tooth to bacterial infection. It can also be indicative of gum disease, an abscess or sinusitis.

What to do

Mild painkillers will deal effectively with the immediate discomfort. Oil of cloves, applied to the affected tooth, is also helpful. However, this should not be used if you are taking homeopathic remedies.

Help!

See a dentist as soon as possible if you experience swelling of any kind – in the gums or face or around the tooth – or if you a running a high temperature. In any case, you should make a dental appointment to find out exactly why you are in pain.

REMEDIES

For immediate treatment of discomfort – **Arnica**

For persistent pain – **Hypericum**

For intense unbearable pain – **Chamomilla**

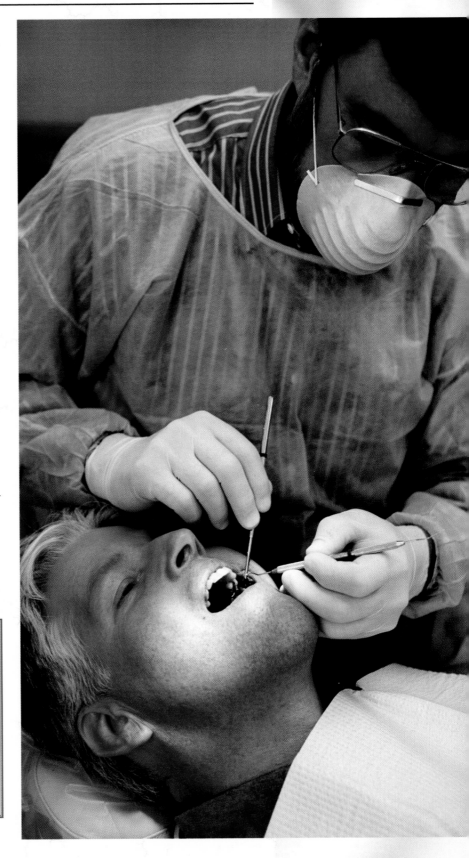

HALITOSIS

Bad breath (halitosis) is a common and embarrassing problem. In itself it can scarcely be classed as a mouth disorder, but it can be a symptom, which should not be ignored.

Causes

Tooth decay is one cause of the problem. Others include gingivitis, indigestion, smoking, tonsillitis, constipation or hunger. Obviously, the consumption of garlic, onions, chilli or similar strong-tasting foods can also be to blame.

What to do

First aid measures for halitosis include scrupulous attention to mouth hygiene, giving up smoking, and avoiding strong-smelling foods. Chewing fresh parsley often helps as a temporary measure.

Below: first aid measures for halitosis include scrupulous attention to mouth hygiene.

Help!

If your gums are bleeding and inflamed, gingivitis is probably the cause of the problem. In severe cases your doctor may prescribe antibiotics. You will also be advised to guard against constipation. If the halitosis is caused by tonsillitis, diabetes, oral thrush or some other serious cause, your doctor will prescribe the appropriate treatment.

REMEDIES

If caused by tooth decay – **Merc. sol.**

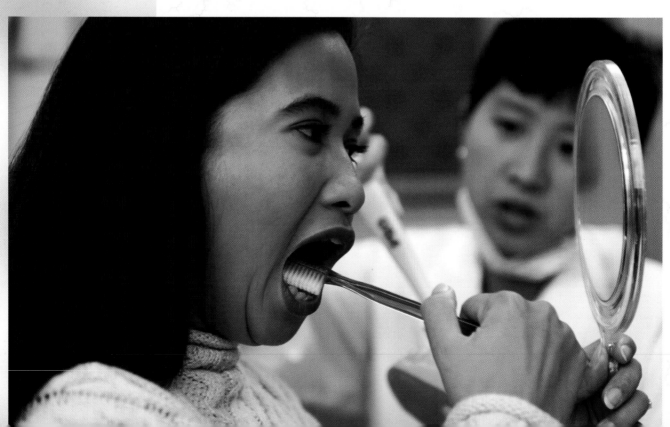

THE SKIN AND HAIR

The skin which, with the hair and nails, comprises the largest organ of the body, accounts for 16% of its total weight. Possible disorders include infections, rashes, allergic reactions and injuries.

Homeopathic practitioners regard skin problems as being indicative of what is happening inside the body.

COMMON PROBLEMS

ACNE

The scourge of the teenage years, acne is a common skin disorder. It creates inflamed red spots on the skin, but can also include blackheads, whiteheads and pustules.

Causes

Acne is often hormone-related. It is caused by an increase in the production of sebum, leading to blocked hair follicles. Over-consumption of sweets and junk food may aggravate the problem. Stress and anxiety, causing excessive sweating, may also be contributory factors.

What to do

The liberal application of medicated soap and hot water, twice daily, is recommended. Squeezing the spots is not. It may cause scars. Get plenty of fresh air, and sunlight in moderation. Avoid fatty, sugary foods. Drink lots of water and eat as much fruit and vegetables as you can.

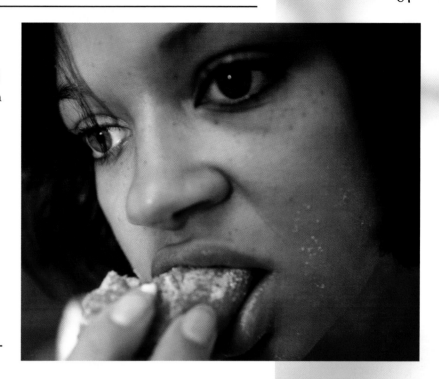

Help!

Acne is not a dangerous complaint, but it gives rise to a great deal of embarrassment and distress at a time when young people are particularly vulnerable. In these circumstances, it is always worthwhile to seek medical advice.

Above: the scourge of the teenage years, acne is a common skin disorder.

REMEDIES

Large painful spots filled with pus – **Hepar. sulph.**

Spots associated with puberty and the onset of menstruation – **Pulsatilla**

Itchy spots on face and shoulders – **Kali. brom.**

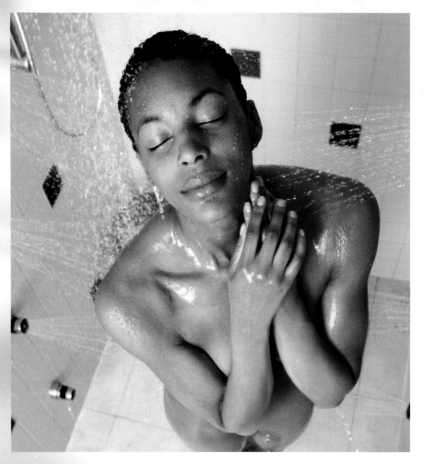

Above: a cool shower may help to alleviate the itching.

What to do

A cool shower may help to alleviate the itching and the application of calamine lotion is sometimes helpful. Resist any temptation to scratch or rub the weals.

Help!

Consult a doctor if there is swelling of the lips or round the eyes.
If there is marked swelling of the throat, call an ambulance at once. In the majority of cases, urticaria disappears within hours and does not require medical treatment.

REMEDIES

Lips and eyelids swollen – **Apis**

For rash caused by stinging nettles – **Urtica**

URTICARIA

Also known as hives or nettle rash, this is an allergic reaction causing raised, itchy red weals on the skin. The weals usually appear on the limbs and the trunk, though in some cases swelling around the lips and the eyes may occur.

Causes

Urticaria is most commonly an allergic reaction, and it is important that the trigger should be found with speed. Triggers may include certain foods, drugs, plants, shellfish, insect bites and excessive heat or cold.

DANDRUFF

Dandruff tends to be at its worst in adolescence, though people of all ages can be affected. It is characterised by an itchy scalp and the production of scales of dry skin. Although this is not a dangerous condition, it is uncomfortable and unsightly.

Causes
Dandruff may be a form of eczema or may be symptomatic of psoriasis or a fungal infection.

What to do
Keep the hair and scalp scrupulously clean, being particularly careful to rinse out all traces of shampoo. Refrain from scratching the scalp, as this may make it bleed and worsen the condition. Gentle head massage may improve the flow of blood and help to alleviate the problem.

Help!
Dandruff does not usually need medical attention and is mainly treated with medicated shampoos. However, if the condition persists or if the scalp becomes inflamed and sore, ask your doctor's advice.

REMEDIES

Scalp is dry, flaky and hot – **Arsen. alb.**

Scalp itches and burns – **Sulphur**

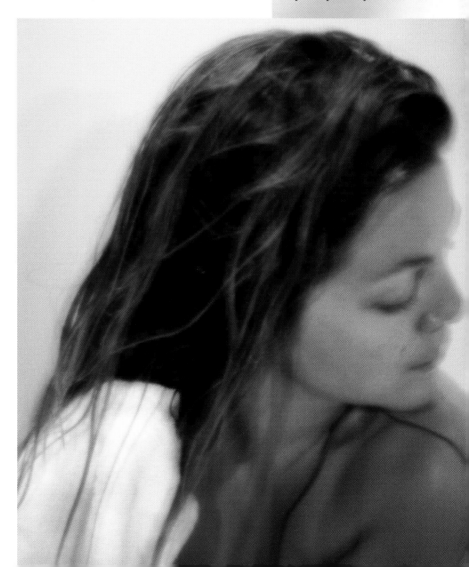

Below: keep the hair and scalp scrupulously clean.

EMOTIONAL PROBLEMS

Both conscious and unconscious bodily functions are controlled by the central nervous system. Although a great deal is known about certain brain functions, the nature of the emotions and the links between the brain and psychiatric problems remain a mystery.

COMMON PROBLEMS

DEPRESSION

There can be few people who do not, from time to time, feel "fed up". Generally, though, this sadness is merely a response to one or another of life's normal events. It should not be confused with true depression that, medically, is a mental illness.

Causes
Depression can be caused by a number of physical problems – an under-active thyroid, a viral infection or chemical imbalance or it may occur after childbirth. Other causes include bereavement or divorce, and redundancy. Depression is often caused by a generally negative attitude resulting in feelings of self-pity, guilt, frustration and loneliness.

What to do
Physical activity, like scrubbing a floor or some heavy gardening, will get your adrenalin flowing and could banish mildly depressed feelings immediately. A social outing may also help.

If you feel the need, discuss your problems with a good friend or even a qualified counsellor. Try a spot of positive thinking, too. The old Emile Coué affirmation 'Every day in every way I am getting better and better,' often works like a charm.

If depression persists for more than a few days, see your doctor.

Help!
Your GP will almost certainly offer some sensible advice about your lifestyle, sleeping and eating habits, and so on. He may also prescribe a short course of anti-depressants or refer you to a psychologist. If there is no improvement in your condition within a fairly short time – three or four weeks – don't hesitate to tell your doctor. Should you be suffering from true clinical depression, he will have further advice to offer.

REMEDIES

Generally low spirits – **China**

After grief or bereavement – **Ignatia**

Tearful, demanding reassurance – **Pulsatilla**

Homeopathic treatment for depression will almost certainly be constitutional and an early consultation with a practitioner is recommended.

INSOMNIA

Insomnia can be defined as the inability to get to sleep or being awake for long periods during the night. As with depression, most people suffer from insomnia from time to time. This problem can result in peevishness, daytime tiredness, headaches and a tendency to tears. It is a fact, though, that these symptoms are often caused not through lack of sleep but because the sufferer has convinced himself that they have not had sufficient rest.

Causes

Sleeplessness is usually caused by stress or worry. Drinking coffee or alcohol just before bedtime can be a contributory factor, as can a heavy meal. Pain or discomfort may cause insomnia and it is also common in old age.

What to do

Many people believe that they need more sleep than is actually the case. That being so, don't worry if you suffer from the occasional sleepless night. However, if the problem persists, take some sensible steps to remedy the situation. Get plenty of exercise during the day. Try to establish a routine of going to bed at the same time every night. Have a warm drink – milk, Horlicks or a herbal tea – before you go to bed. Ensure that the bedroom is airy but comfortably warm.

Help!

There is no need to consult a doctor about occasional insomnia, but if it persists ask your GP for advice. If your sleeplessness is caused by pain or illness, they will obviously address the problem. However, they are unlikely to suggest sleep-inducing drugs, as these can be addictive.

REMEDIES

Sudden onset of insomnia – **Coffea**

Irritability as a result of insomnia – **Nux vomica**

Tired but unable to sleep – **Opium**

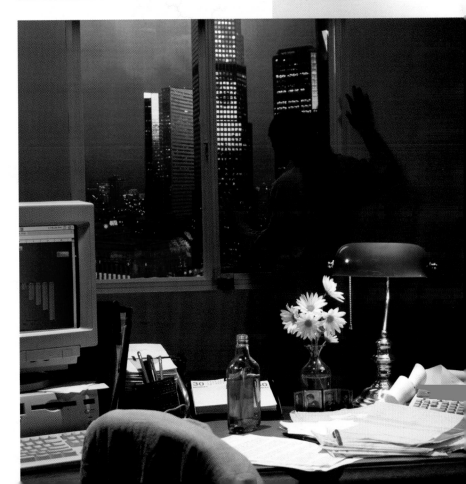

Below: insomnia can be defined as the inability to get to sleep or being awake for long periods during the night.

TREATING OTHER PEOPLE

As your family and friends learn of your interest in homeopathy and notice the success of your self-treatment, they will start to regard you as something of an oracle. They'll soon realise, too, that getting a homeopathic prescription from you is easier than waiting for an hour in the GP's surgery. As a result, you are likely to be besieged by people seeking a magical cure. In the beginning, at any rate, it would be unwise to accede to these demands.

1 First – you lack the necessary experience.

2 Second – a remedy that works well for you may be useless for another person who has a completely different psychological make-up.

3 Third – the would-be patient may not provide you with the essential explicit details of their problems.

Sometimes, these details will be held back because they embarrass the patient. At other times, they may consider them too trivial to mention. It must be clearly understood that withholding such details – whatever the reason for doing so – can radically affect the accuracy of the homeopathic prescription.

Safety measures

However successfully you may have treated your own ailments, be wary of prescribing for other people. Always remember that homeopathy treats the whole person. No matter how close your relationship with relatives or friends, there are almost sure to be facets of their lives or personalities of which you are unaware. Until you have gained a fair amount of experience in homeopathy, don't be persuaded into prescribing for them.

Right: however successfully you may have treated your own ailments, be wary of prescribing for other people.

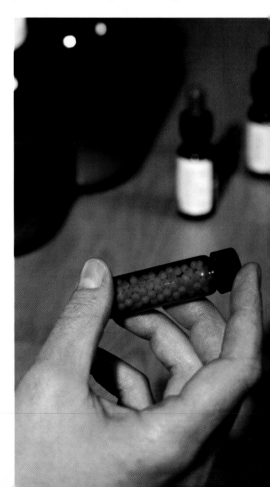

DANGER SIGNALS

By all means, reassure them if they are agitated and help them to list their symptoms. Some of these symptoms should act as danger signals. If they occur, your sole intervention should be in advising the patient to take immediate action. Call an ambulance or send for a doctor if the patient has:

Severe pain in the chest or arms

Breathing problems

Serious abdominal pain

Coughing up of blood

Persistent/unexplained giddiness or vertigo

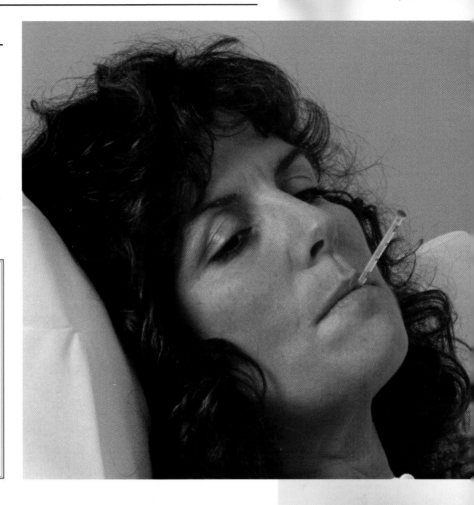

Above: danger signals require speedy medical attention.

Other symptoms requiring speedy medical attention include a long-standing sore throat or cough, tiredness, weight loss, persistent severe headaches, visual disturbances, back pain, unexplained swelling in any part of the body, blood in urine or faeces and changes in bladder or bowel habits.

If the would-be patient complains of any of these symptoms, recommend that they should make an urgent appointment with their medical advisor. Don't be tempted to prescribe anything.

Homeopathy, in itself, is absolutely safe. The danger lies in the possibility that a remedy may seem to alleviate serious symptoms and thereby allow the condition to worsen because medical attention is not sought.

It is important to remember that you, too, should be alert for any of these danger signals when prescribing for yourself.

HOMEOPATHY FOR CHILDREN

Childhood ailments are rarely serious, but can be distressing for both parent and patient, particularly if the child happens to be your first-born and you lack experience of the ups and downs of parenthood. Homeopathy comes into its own here, providing gentle, natural remedies with no risk of the side-effects so common with conventional drugs.

What's more, homeopathic treatment is easily administered and, by fostering the child's natural resistance to illness, can ensure a speedy recovery.

Childhood is usually considered to cover the period from twelve months to twelve years of age. Illnesses experienced during this time help to develop the body's in-built immunity to disease and can therefore have a decisive effect on health in later life.

As always, you should consult a conventional doctor if your child appears to be seriously ill or if, after homeopathic treatment, the condition fails to improve. However, most childish ailments will respond swiftly to homeopathic remedies.

This is particularly true of the more common problems of the early years. That being so, you would be well advised to arm yourself with a reliable reference book (see Appendix) and a small supply of "stand by" remedies.

ACONITE
ARNICA
ARSEN. ALB.
BELLADONNA
BRYONIA
FERRUM PHOS.
GELSEMIUM
HEPAR. SULPH.
NUX VOMICA
PHOSPHOROUS
PULSATILLA
RHUS TOX.

You will find that some of the remedies mentioned above are also included in the recommended homeopathic first aid box (see page 83) It is sensible to duplicate where necessary, so that you can keep the children's remedies readily to hand.

NB: Keep them safely away from the hands of your inquisitive offspring.

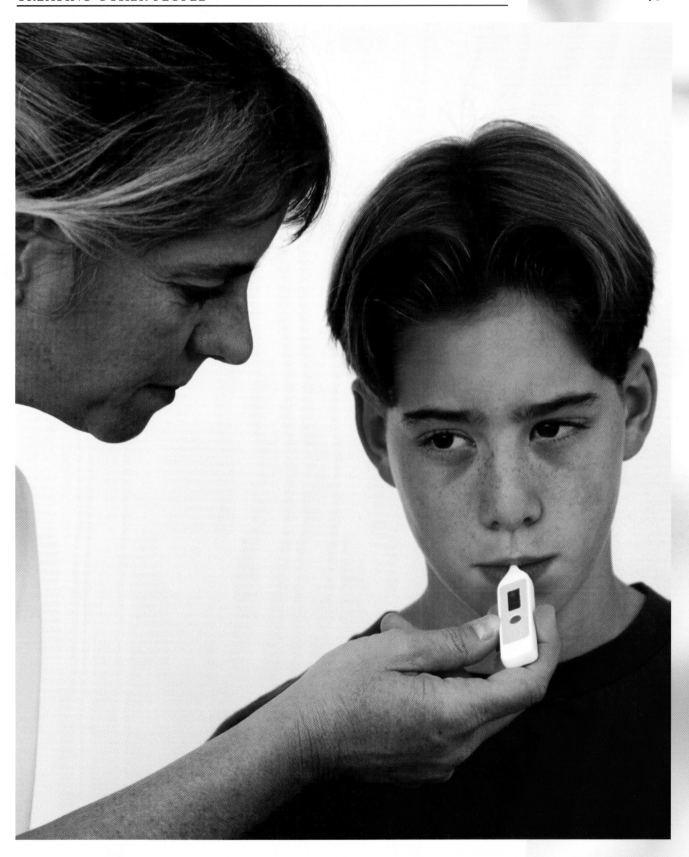

PROBLEMS WITH PUBERTY

Dealing with adolescents is never easy. The hormones are in a state of flux, producing profound physical and emotional effects in youngsters of both sexes.

At an extremely vulnerable time in their lives, teenagers are caught up in a maelstrom of change. Boys, already self-consciously aware of enlargement of the genitals and the sudden appearance of bodily hair, are further embarrassed by a voice that varies abruptly between soprano and baritone. Girls are faced with the onset of menstruation, the appearance of bodily hair in the armpits and around the genitals, and with the development of breasts. And, of course, both sexes suffer from that scourge of the teenage years – acne (see page 67).

Parents, trying to help their children through these difficult years, must also contend with two more powerful influences – peer pressure and media power. In fact, you may find you need homeopathic help yourself to alleviate the strain of coping with recalcitrant teenagers.

Homeopathy can offer support and comfort to all concerned. During periods of academic stress or emotional upheavals, long-term homeopathic treatment may be indicated. At such times, it is always wise to seek a consultation with a professional homeopathic practitioner who will be able to define your child's constitutional type.

However, many of the upsets of the teenage years can be alleviated by homeopathic self-help. Remedies suggested in addition to those in the first aid kit include:

Below: at an extremely vulnerable time in their lives, teenagers are caught up in a maelstrom of change.

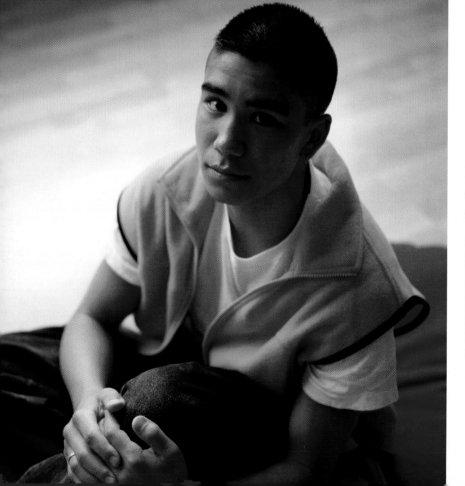

For body odour – **Calc. carb. or Merc. sol.**

For examination nerves – **Argent. nit.** *or* **Anacardium occ.**

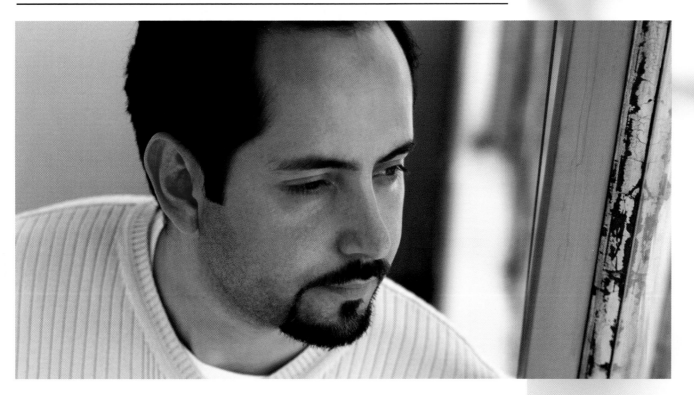

HOMEOPATHY FOR MEN

Men, it is said, are the stronger sex. It is true that their physical make-up is less complicated than that of women. Many of the problems from which they suffer are the result of infection, ranging from head colds to disorders of the reproductive system.

Most men are reluctant to seek medical help, particularly for problems with the reproductive system. Usually, such conditions are easily treated, but prompt action is necessary to avoid the development of complications.

Because homeopathic remedies are particularly effective in dealing with infections, they offer a quick and

convenient form of self-treatment for most male problems. Self-treatment, too, spares the embarrassed male the ordeal of discussing the situation with his doctor.

Suggestions are given below for simple homeopathic remedies that will deal effectively with many male problems.

> *For erectile dysfunction –* **Conium or Agnus**
>
> *For thrush –* **Merc. sol.**
>
> *NB: If any symptoms persist for five days, a doctor should be consulted.*

Above: most men are reluctant to seek medical help.

HOMEOPATHY FOR WOMEN

Many of the health problems suffered by women are linked to the reproductive system, beginning with the onset of menstruation and continuing to the menopause. Obviously, hormone levels are much involved. Because homeopathy is an holistic therapy, it is particularly effective in dealing with women's complaints.

Below: because homeopathy is an holistic therapy, it is particularly effective in dealing with women's complaints.

If you, as a woman, intend to self-prescribe homeopathic remedies it is particularly important that you should first ascertain your constitutional type. Asking help from friends and family will not help.

Their answers will be influenced by their own perceptions and their relationship with you. A consultation with a professional homeopath will provide the information you need and be well worthwhile.

Suggestions for dealing with some of the most common women's ailments include:

For Premenstrual Syndrome (PMS) – **Sepia** and/or **Nat. mur.**

For heavy periods – **Nux vomica** or **Belladonna**

For breast pain – **Conium** and/or **Bryonia**

For hot flushes – **Amyl nit.**

For cystitis – **Cantharis**

NB: These remedies may be regarded as "standard" suggestions for the problems mentioned. Depending on the patient's constitutional type, other prescriptions may be are more helpful.

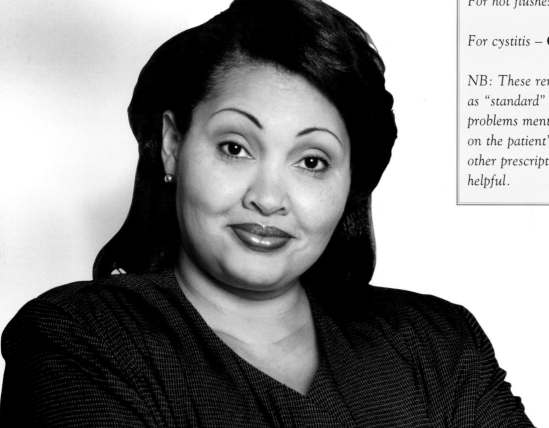

HOMEOPATHY FOR THE ELDERLY

Frequent references are made in the media to the increasing number of over-60s in the population. Undoubtedly, people are living longer. It is obviously important, therefore, that they should maintain good health for as long as possible.

It is an inescapable fact that physical and mental capacities tend to deteriorate with age. Even so, much can be done to lessen the impact of advancing years and to slow down the onset of age-related problems.

A positive, upbeat approach to life is valuable in maintaining vitality at any age. Long-term use of homeopathy can correct systemic imbalances. Furthermore, the gentle, natural action of homeopathic remedies is better suited to elderly people who may find the side-effects of conventional drugs difficult to cope with.

A sensible, nutritious diet, gentle exercise in the fresh air and sufficient rest are of primary importance for the maintenance of good health in elderly people. In addition, it makes sense to keep in hand a few homeopathic remedies for dealing with any of the common problems most likely to arise.

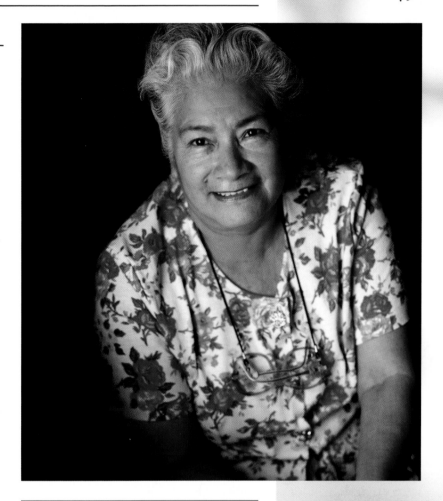

Above: it is an inescapable fact that physical and mental capacities tend to deteriorate with age

*For bladder incontinence – **Causticum***

*After a fall – **Arnica***

*For bruising – **Arnica ointment***

*For dizzy spells – **Theridion***

*For confusion – **Baryta carb.***

NB: *It is important not to take risks with any situation that may arise with elderly people. It is safe to give the remedies suggested here, but if the condition is not quickly resolved, call a doctor.*

ACCIDENTS AND EMERGENCIES

No matter how great your faith in homeopathic remedies, it's unlikely that you will have them to hand outside the home. If an accident happens in a shop, in the street or in any other public place, the emergency services usually arrive with speed. You are unlikely to be involved, beyond perhaps comforting the patient until help arrives.

Below: if an accident happens in a shop, in the street or in any other public place, the emergency services usually arrive with speed.

Crises that occur in the home or garden are another matter. Sometimes, homeopathic treatment is all that is needed. Even so, you must not allow your enthusiasm to run away with you.

Stay calm

Whatever the emergency – stay calm. Your first action must be to establish priorities. Determine exactly what has happened. How severe is the problem? Check on the following essential points.

> *Is the patient's breathing laboured or non-existent?*
>
> *Is the patient badly injured?*
>
> *Is the patient bleeding profusely?*
>
> *Are any bones broken?*
>
> *Is the patient badly burned?*
>
> *Is the patient in a state of severe shock?*

If the answer to any of these questions is "yes", you should call an ambulance immediately.

Reassure the patient that help is on the way. Keep a watchful eye for any worsening of their condition. If possible, place them in the recovery position (see illustration). Keep them as warm as possible.

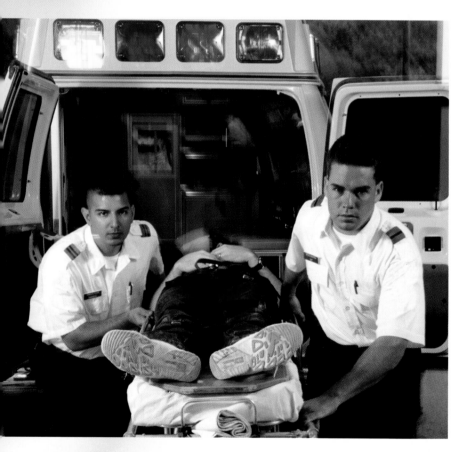

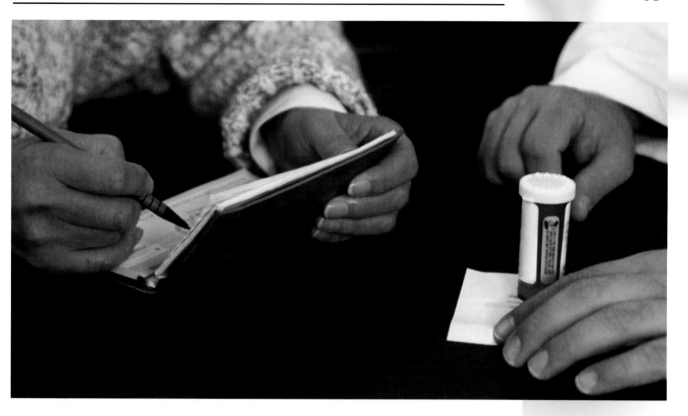

First aid

Once you become involved with homeopathic self-treatment, you will probably want to keep a small supply of remedies in the house. At this point, perhaps we should look at those problems that most commonly arise in a home situation and consider the most useful remedies.

Asthma attacks

If the patient is using conventional medicine, prescribed by a doctor, you should on no account suggest that this is discontinued. Drosera may help to calm the patient's anxiety and to relieve the breathing problems. Ipecacuanha is particularly useful when the patient is suffering from a great deal of phlegm.

Anxiety

Anxiety arises from a variety of situations and can often involve deep depression. A generally nervous attitude responds well to Gelsemium. Arsenicum will help when the patient is fearful and exhausted.

Bereavement

Sudden bereavement always comes as a shock. Ignatia is effective in treating the initial impact. If a storm of weeping results, Pulsatilla will help, but Nat. mur. is the remedy for repressed grief, where the patient seems numb and unable to comprehend what has happened.

Above: once you become involved with homeopathic self-treatment, you will probably want to keep a small supply of remedies in the house.

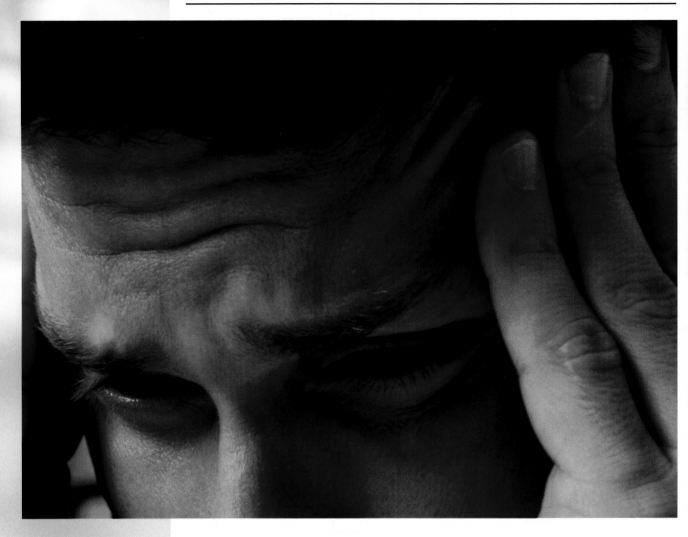

Above: homeopathy is particularly well equipped to deal with stress.

Burns
Don't attempt to treat large burns. Small burns should be immersed in cold water, then covered with cling film or a special burn dressing. On no account should you apply anything to the burn, but Arnica, taken in tablet form, will help to alleviate the pain.

Nosebleed
Both Arnica and Phosphorous tablets are helpful but, if the bleeding persists for 20 minutes or more, consult your GP.

Stress
Any of the above conditions – and many others – can cause stress. Homeopathy is particularly well equipped to deal with this. Ledum may be prescribed when the stressed person is angry and resentful. If the condition is caused by over-exertion and consequent lack of energy, Carbo veg. will help.

YOUR FIRST AID BOX

You will need about 10 basic remedies in your first aid kit. This should include ointments and tinctures as well as tablets. Among the most commonly used remedies are:

Arnica

This remedy, in tablet form, is excellent for dealing with shock. Arnica ointment swiftly reduces swelling and lessens the pain of bruising.

Aconite

When symptoms such as colds and flu suddenly appear, Aconite acts as a sedative and analgesic. It is also useful for dealing with any form of emotional stress, including panic attacks.

Carbo veg. (charcoal)

The use of charcoal as a digestive remedy dates back many years. It will reduce bloating, flatulence and heartburn and is also effective in dealing with headaches produced by over-eating.

Apis

This remedy is a perfect example of like curing like. Produced from whole bees, including the sting, it deals with inflammation, the burning, stinging pain produced by cystitis, nettle rash and insect bites.

Hypericum

Commonly known as St John's Wort, this treatment has soared in popularity as a treatment for depression. The tablets are also effective in reducing nerve or back pain. Hypericum cream or tincture will deal with grazes and painful wounds.

In addition to these five basic remedies, your first aid box should also contain tinctures and ointments. We suggest:

Tinctures

These are used, diluted in cool boiled water, for cleansing wounds. Use 10 drops of the chosen tincture to 1.25 litres of water.

your first aid box should Include:

Arnica

Calendula

Euphrasia

Hypericum

Ointments

Homeopathic ointments and creams are particularly effective in soothing pain. They also promote healing and protect the wound against infection.

Your first aid box should include:

Arnica ointment*

Calendula cream

Hypericum ointment

Urtica ointment

*Do not apply arnica ointment if the skin is broken.

More useful remedies

The remedies listed above form a basic homeopathic first aid kit, but useful additions include Belladonna, Bryonia, Cantharis, Chamomilla, Hepar. sulph., Magnesium phos., Nux vomica and Ruta. As your experience grows, you will undoubtedly find other favourite remedies you will wish to add.

Other equipment

You will, of course, include in your kit the usual basic items required for any form of first aid, such as sterile pads, adhesive dressings, cotton wool, etc. All of these can be readily obtained from any pharmacy.

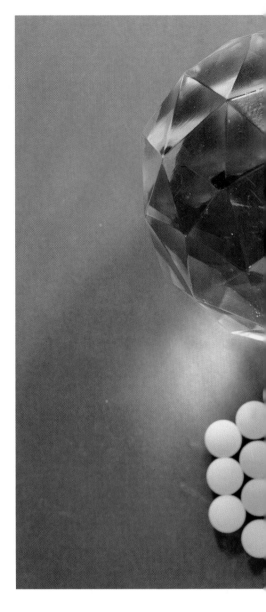

Note, too, that some pharmacies sell complete homeopathic first aid kits. These provide a good start, but you should check that the remedies you require are included. Check, too, that instructions for use of all over-the-counter remedies are provided. Follow these precisely. If in doubt, consult a homeopathic directory.

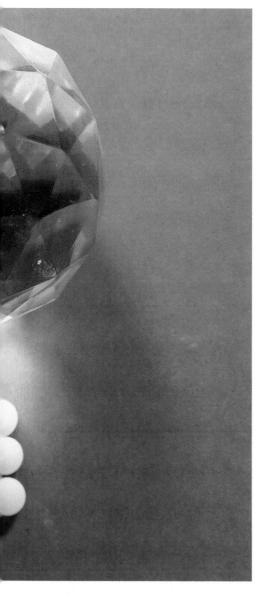

BIOCHEMIC TISSUE SALTS

Biochemic tissue salts differ from other homeopathic remedies in that they are prepared only from minerals, such as rock salt and quartz. The principle of the minimum dose is followed and the salts are prepared in the same way as homeopathic remedies.

The salts were developed by a German homeopathic doctor, Wilhelm Schuessler. In 1873 he published a treatise claiming that

many diseases were caused by a deficiency of certain inorganic minerals in the body. He claimed that lack of a particular mineral would produce specific symptoms. His theory was that the illness could be cured by a minute dose of the tissue salt containing the missing mineral.

Like most homeopathic remedies, tissue salts are produced as tiny lactose tablets. There are only 12 varieties:

Left: biochemic tissue salts differ from other homeopathic remedies in that they are prepared only from minerals, such as rock salt and quartz.

Storage

Find a clean wooden box in which to keep your first aid items and store it somewhere cool, dark, dry and easily accessible. Tell all adult members of your household where the box is kept, but keep it well out of the reach of children. Correctly stored, homeopathic remedies can be kept indefinitely without loss of strength.

Calc. fluor. (Calcium fluoride) prescribed for circulatory problems, varicose veins, haemorrhoids and dental problems.

Calc. phos. (Calcium phosphate) prescribed for under-nourished states, indigestion, chilblains, colds and catarrh.

Calc. sulph. (Calcium sulphate) prescribed for skin ailments, slow healing, headaches, neuralgia and kidney problems.

Ferrum phos. (Iron phosphate) prescribed for rheumatism, haemor- rhages, respiratory problems and feverish conditions.

Kali. mur. (Potassium chloride) prescribed for catarrh, ear infections, congested conditions and thick white discharges.

Kali. phos. (Potassium phosphate) prescribed for nervous tension, depression, headaches, incontinence and shyness.

Below: homeopathic tablets.

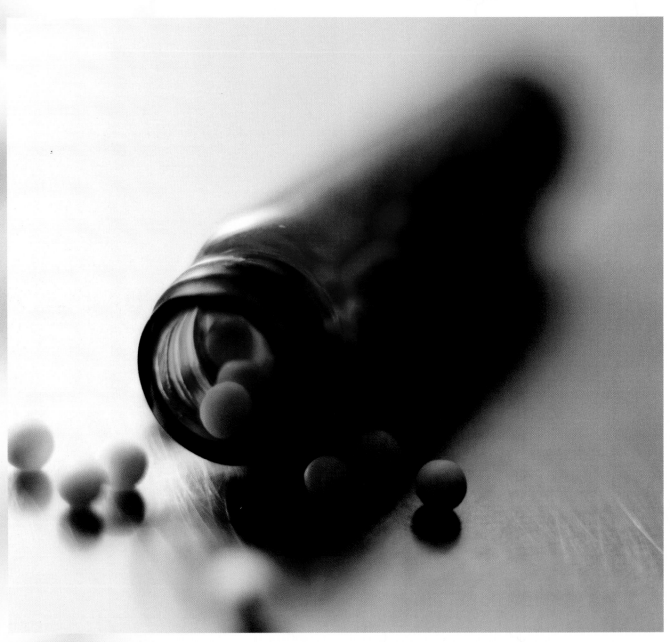

Kali. sulph. (Potassium sulphate) prescribed for skin ailments, catarrh, palpitations, menstrual problems and halitosis.

Mag. phos. (Magnesium phosphate) prescribed for cramp, flatulence, hiccups, menstrual pain and neuralgia.

Nat. mur. (Sodium chloride) prescribed for cold sores, mouth ulcers, depression, dryness or excessive moisture in any part of the body.

Nat. phos. (Sodium phosphate) prescribed for acidity, stomach upsets, heartburn, constipation, diarrhoea and nausea.

Nat. sulph. (Sodium sulphate) prescribed for hay fever, digestive problems, water retention and liver upsets.

Silica (Silicon dioxide) prescribed for boils, styes, nail problems, neurological disorders and lack of vitality.

Combination remedies
Eighteen combined tissue salt remedies, designated by letters of the alphabet, are now available, specially formulated for use with certain groups of ailments.

As with the single tissue salts, the combinations are marketed in small tubs, each containing information about the ailments covered and the precise dosage. These are sold at most pharmacies and health food shops.

Do they work?
Biochemic tissue salts are widely used by homeopathic practitioners. Some doctors prescribe them, though there have been insufficient clinical trials to establish their value. They are widely used in the self-treatment of various minor ailments and, as with homeopathic remedies, the tablets are harmless.

More information
If you are interested in using the tissue salts, you will find plenty of guidance in several small books published over the past few years (see Appendix).

Although biochemistry and homeopathy have much in common, they are in fact quite distinct branches of medicine. Nonetheless, all the 12 tissue salts recommended by Dr Schuessler are also used in homeopathic remedies.

QUICK REFERENCE GUIDE

This section contains a quick reference guide to the homeopathic remedies mentioned in this book, together with brief details of their recommended use.

This guide should be regarded as your initial resource. Always consult a more comprehensive reference book before deciding on remedies for yourself or for other people.

ACONITE
Acute respiratory infections, coughs, colds

AGNUS
Fatigue, postnatal depression

AMMONIUM MUR.
Liver problems, respiratory disorders, sciatica

AMYL NIT.
Chest pains, hot flushes, menopausal symptoms

ANACARDIUM OCC.
Examination nerves, spots, teenage problems

APIS
Stings and insect bites, urticaria

ARGENT. NIT.
Fears and phobias, diarrhoea, vertigo, IBS

ARSEN. ALB.
Food poisoning, digestive problems, headaches

BARYTA CARB.
Respiratory problems, impotence, anxiety

BELLADONNA
Feverish conditions, headaches, migraine

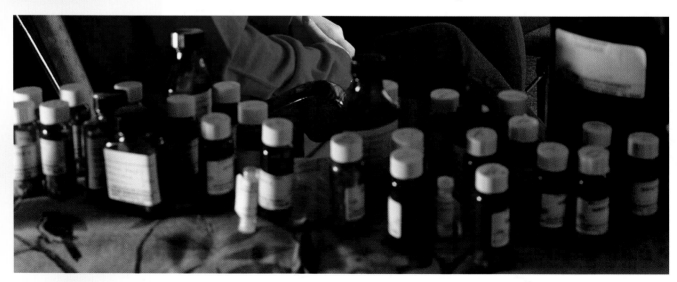

BERBERIS
Kidney problems, cystitis, pain in lower back

BRYONIA
Dry coughs, constipation, colds and influenza

CACTUS
Angina, muscular pain and constriction

CALC. CARB.
Problems with joint, bones and teeth, women's ailments

CALENDULA
Cuts, injuries, varicose ulcers, blisters

CANTHARIS
Bladder infections, cystitis, burns and scalds, insect bites

CARBO VEG.
Digestive problems, flatulence, breathing difficulties

CARBON SULPH.
Sciatic pain, skin irritation, digestive problems, tinnitus

CAUSTICUM
Coughs, skin problems, urinary disorders

CHAMOMILLA
Helps teething babies, menstrual pain, colic and diarrhoea

CHINA
Insomnia, headaches, feverish conditions

CHINA SULPH.
Tinnitus, pains in joints, severe head pain

COFFEA
Nerves, hot flushes in menopause, palpitations

COLOCYNTHIS
Spasmodic pain, diarrhoea, menstrual problems

CONIUM
Prostate problems, sexual difficulties, nervous conditions

CUPRUM MET.
Coughs, exhaustion, stomach pains, asthma

DROSERA
Spasmodic cough, whooping cough, restlessness, vomiting

EUPHRASIA
Conjunctivitis, hay fever, colds

FERRUM MET.
Anaemia, headaches, fatigue, digestive problems

GELSEMIUM
Influenza, nervous exhaustion, hay fever, exam. nerves, stage fright

GRAPHITES
Anxiety, erectile difficulties, menstrual problems

HAMAMELIS
Varicose veins, nosebleeds, heavy menstruation

HEPAR. SULPH.
Acne, colds, coughs, catarrh, sore throat

HYPERICUM
Nerve injuries, concussion, toothache, depression

IGNATIA
Emotional problems, insomnia, headaches, grief

IPECACUANHA
Asthma, nausea, coughs, menstrual problems

KALI. BROM.
Male sexual difficulties, mental problems, skin problems

KALI. CARB.
Incontinence, kidney problems, palpitations, coughs

KALI. PHOS.
Perspiration, insomnia, discharges, fatigue

LACHESIS
PMS and menopausal symptoms, varicose veins, heart problems

LATRODECTUS
Angina, restlessness

LEDUM
Black eyes and similar injuries, insect stings, open wounds

LYCOPODIUM
Distension, wind, digestive discomfort, anxiety

MAGNESIUM PHOS.
Menstrual cramps relieved by warmth, colic, neuralgia

MERC. SOL.
Toothache, earache, fever, osteoarthritis

NAJA
Angina, palpitations, erratic pulse

NAT. MUR.
Skin conditions, digestive problems, headaches

NUX VOMICA
Hangovers, constipation, PMS, insomnia

OPIUM
Constipation, shock, injury, grief

PAEONIA
Nightmares, rectal and anal problems

PHOSPHOROUS
Bleeding, cough, palpitations, respiratory problems

PULSATILLA
Ear troubles, colds, eye infections, female disorders

RHUS TOX.
Rheumatic or arthritic pain, sprains, backache, bladder problems

RUTA
Injuries to joints, arthritis, eyestrain, sciatica

SEPIA
Female disorders, skin conditions, digestive problems

SILICA
Diabetes, boils, abscesses, constipation, digestive problems

STAPHISAGRIA
Styes, insomnia, joint pains, cystitis

SULPHUR
Men's health, digestive problems, respiratory disorders

THERIDION
Diabetes, acute sensitivity of the bones, nerves and spine

URTICA
Rashes, blistering, urticaria

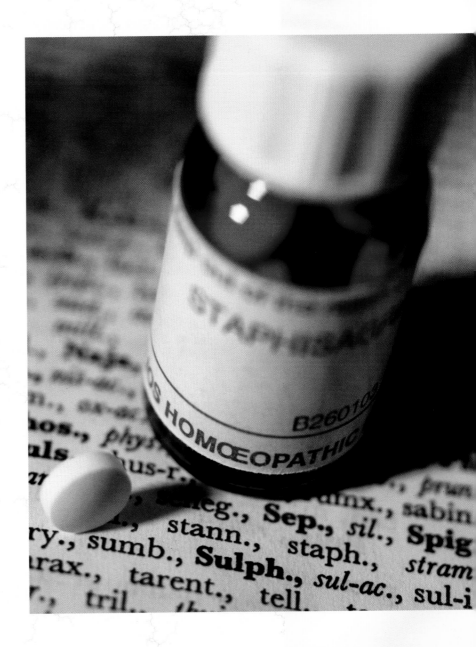

USEFUL ADDRESSES AN FURTHER READING

Professional organisations:

The British Homeopathic
Association
27a Devonshire Street,
London W1N 1RJ

The Society of Homeopaths
2 Artizan Road,
Northampton NN1 4HU

Faculty of Homeopathy
15 Clerkenwell Close,
London EC1R 0AA

**Suppliers of homeopathic
remedies:**

Nelson and Co. Ltd.
5 Endeavour Way,
London SW19 9UH

Weleda (UK) Ltd.
Heanor Road, Ilkeston,
Derbyshire DE7 8DR

Homeopathic hospitals:

Royal London Homeopathic Hospital
Great Ormond Street,
London WC1N 3HR

Glasgow Homeopathic Hospital
1053 Great Western Road,
Glasgow G12 0XQ

Tunbridge Wells Homeopathic
Hospital
Church Road, Tunbridge Wells,
Kent TN1 1JU

**The Complete Family Guide to
Homeopathy**
Dr Christopher Hammond
Element Books Ltd

Encyclopedia of Homeopathy
Dr Andrew Lockie
Dorling Kindersley

**Homeopathy: Medicine of the
New Man**
George Vithoulkas
Thorsons

**Homeopathy: for Babies and
Children**
Beth MacEoin
Headway – Hodder & Stoughton

Homeopathy
Keith A. Scott and Linda A. McCourt
Thorsons

**Natural Therapies: What They
Are: What They Do**
Mark Evans and Sebastian Kelly

**The Complete Guide to Integrated
Medicine**
Dr David Peters and Anne Woodham
Dorling Kindersley

Doctor, What's the Alternative?
Dr Hilary Jones
Hodder & Stoughton

Biochemic Handbook
J.S. Goodwin
Thorsons

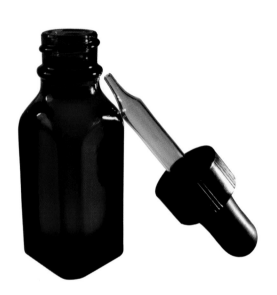